Pocket Primer for Nutritional Health

Norman J. Temple • Ted Wilson
Editors

Pocket Primer for Nutritional Health

Springer

Editors
Norman J. Temple
Centre for Science
Athabasca University
Athabasca, AB, Canada

Ted Wilson
Department of Biology
Winona State University
Winona, MN, USA

ISBN 978-3-032-25401-6 ISBN 978-3-032-25402-3 (eBook)
https://doi.org/10.1007/978-3-032-25402-3

This Springer imprint is published by the registered company Springer Nature Switzerland AG
The registered company address is: Gewerbestrasse 11, 6330 Cham, Switzerland

Preface

A great many advances in our understanding of nutrition took place during the first half of the twentieth century. The focus was largely on vitamins and minerals. Since the 1970s, there has been a flood of research studies on the role of diet in noncommunicable diseases such as obesity, heart disease, and cancer. Today, we have a vastly greater understanding of the role of diet in causing these diseases. We now know, for example, that such foods as whole grain cereals, fruit, vegetables, sugar, and the kinds of meats eaten profoundly affect the risk of developing a wide variety of noncommunicable diseases. This evidence convincingly demonstrates that nutrition serves as an essential weapon in the battle against disease and for the enhancement of human health.

But progress in the field of nutrition has not slowed down. Research findings in the twenty-first century have built on those from the last century and have provided a treasure trove of new information. The focus of this book is topics where advances have been made that are, potentially, of major importance. This takes the form of each chapter providing a brief review of a particular topic.

Topics covered include the following:

- *Obesity*. This includes the causes of the obesity epidemic with a close look taken at ultra-processed food. The chapter includes not only dietary treatments for weight control but also effective treatments that use surgery and drugs.
- *Coronary heart disease*. The evidence that has appeared over recent years has revealed that a generally healthy diet is far more effective for the prevention of heart disease than is a reduction in intake of saturated fats.
- *Ultra-processed food*. The chapter critically evaluates the evidence regarding the impact of these foods on health and disease. Close attention is paid to the relationship between ultra-processed foods and obesity.
- *Healthy alternatives to the Western diet*. This chapter examines various diets that have been proposed as being nutritionally superior to the Western diet. Diets discussed include the Mediterranean diet, the DASH diet, vegetarian diets, and the Planetary Health Diet.
- *Phytochemicals*. An overview is presented on the major types of phytochemicals and the evidence that indicates that these substances enhance health and prevent various diseases.

- *Health promotion.* Health promotion campaigns that provide education and advice to people in order to persuade them to adopt a healthier lifestyle. An alternative strategy is based on government policies. This chapter argues that government policy approaches have been far more successful.
- *Front-of-pack food labels.* The chapter examines various designs for front-of-pack food labels and discusses their effectiveness as tools for encouraging consumers to select healthier foods.
- *Genomics including genomic medicine and personalized nutrition.* Genomic medicine may allow for more accurate predictions of an individual's risk of different diseases. This research may also lead to dietary advice that is tailored to a person's genetics (gene-based personalized nutrition).
- *Microbiome.* The focus of the chapter is the microorganisms present in the colon. The microbiome is believed to have a significant impact on health. The diet appears to have a strong influence on the balance of microorganisms within the microbiome.
- *Sustainable diets.* The widespread adoption of sustainable diets is of great importance because modern agriculture uses enormous amounts of land and natural resources and is a major contributor to climate change. Key features of sustainable diets include a shift toward a plant-based diet, a reduction in food waste, limiting the consumption of ultra-processed foods, utilizing local food systems, and choosing sustainable seafood.
- *Food industry.* This chapter examines how the food industry uses its enormous marketing power to encourage the population to consume unhealthy but profitable foods.

It is undeniable that the population of the planet is living longer, but not always healthier. It is also undeniable that a better understanding of nutrition, especially of recent developments, is critically important for clarification of the misunderstandings that plague the science of nutrition. The goal of this pocket primer is to provide readers with the most important developments in nutrition.

Athabasca, AB, Canada — Norman J. Temple
Winona, MN, USA — Ted Wilson

Contents

1 **Methods in Nutrition Research** 1
David R. Jacobs Jr and Norman J. Temple

2 **Obesity: A Disease of Overnutrition** 15
Catherine M. Champagne and George A. Bray

3 **Coronary Heart Disease, Cardiovascular Disease, and the Role of Diet** 25
Norman J. Temple

4 **Ultra-Processed Foods: Their Impact on Health** 37
Norman J. Temple

5 **Healthier Alternatives to the Western Diet** 47
Jasmine Chen and Karen Davison

6 **Dietary Supplements: What Can Be Recommended?** 63
Norman J. Temple

7 **Phytochemicals in Food and Their Health Benefits** 71
Rafik Assabgui and Karen Davison

8 **Food Synergy: A Paradigm Shift in Nutrition Science** 85
David R. Jacobs Jr and Norman J. Temple

9 **Health Promotion and the Importance of Government Policy** 93
Norman J. Temple

10 **Front-of-Package Food Labels: Their Types, History, Impact on Consumer Behavior, and Support by Digital Technologies** 105
Nikola Ljusic

11 **Genomics Medicine and Personalized Nutrition** 117
Ashwini Rajasekaran, Jasmine Chen, and Karen Davison

12 **Nutritional Health and the Microbiome** 129
Allison L. Brichacek, Katherine A. Maki, and Nicole Farmer

13 Diets for Sustainable Food Systems ... 145
Andrew Berardy and Joan Sabaté

14 Industry Influence: The Food Environment and Nutrition Policy ... 157
Julia McCarthy

15 An Overview of Key Advances in Nutrition: More Than the Sum of the Parts ... 167
Norman J. Temple and Karen Davison

Appendices ... 183

Index ... 191

Editors and Contributors

About the Editors

Norman J. Temple, PhD was the Professor of Nutrition at Athabasca University in Alberta, Canada. He is now a Professor Emeritus. He has published 100 papers, mainly in the area of nutrition in relation to health. He has also published 14 books. Together with Denis Burkitt he coedited *Western Diseases: Their Dietary Prevention and Reversibility* (1994). This continued and extended Burkitt's pioneering work on the role of dietary fiber in chronic diseases of lifestyle. He coedited *Nutritional Health: Strategies for Disease Prevention* (2023; fourth edition), *Nutrition Guide for Physicians and Related Healthcare Professions* (2022; third edition), *Beverage Impacts on Health and Nutrition* (2016; second edition), *Community Nutrition for Developing Countries* (2016), and *Excessive Medical Spending: Facing the Challenge* (2007). He has conducted collaborative research in Cape Town on the role of the changing diet in South Africa on the pattern of diseases in that country, such as obesity, diabetes, and heart disease.

Ted Wilson, PhD is Professor of Biology at Winona State University in Winona, Minnesota. His research examines how diet affects human nutritional physiology and whether food/dietary supplement health claims can be supported by measurable physiological changes. He has studied many foods, dietary supplements, and disease conditions including walnuts, pistachios, low-carbohydrate diets, cranberries, cranberry juice, apple juice, grape juice, wine, resveratrol, creatine phosphate, soy phytoestrogens, eggplants, coffee, tea, energy drinks, heart failure prognosis, diabetes, and obesity. Diet-induced changes have included physiological evaluations of plasma lipid profile, antioxidants, vasodilation, nitric oxide, platelet aggregation, and glycemic and insulinemic responses using in vivo and in vitro models. With Dr. N. Temple he edited *Nutritional Health: Strategies for Disease Prevention*, *Nutrition Guide for Physicians*, and *Beverages in Nutrition and Health*. He also enjoys teaching courses in Nutrition, Physiology, Cardiovascular Physiology, Cell Signal Transduction, and Cell Biology. When not working in the laboratory, he enjoys family time, the outdoors, and farming.

Contributors

Rafik Assabgui Agriculture and Agri-Food Canada, Ottawa, ON, Canada

Andrew Berardy Department of Geography & Earth Sciences, United States Military Academy, West Point, NY, USA

George A. Bray Pennington Biomedical Research Center, Baton Rouge, LA, USA

Allison L. Brichacek Department of Laboratory Medicine, National Institutes of Health Clinical Center, Bethesda, MD, USA

Catherine M. Champagne Pennington Biomedical Research Center, Baton Rouge, LA, USA

Jasmine Chen Department of Public Health and Social Policy, University of Victoria, Victoria, BC, Canada

Karen Davison Institute for Life Course and Aging, University of Toronto & The Centre of Clinical Excellence, Toronto, ON, Canada

Centre for Science, Athabasca University, Athabasca, AB, Canada

Nicole Farmer Translational Biobehavioral and Health Promotion Branch, National Institutes of Health Clinical Center, Bethesda, MD, USA

David R. Jacobs Jr. Division of Epidemiology and Community Health, School of Public Health, University of Minnesota, Minneapolis, MN, USA

Nikola Ljusic Behavior and Technology Lab, Kristiania University of Applied Sciences, Oslo, Norway

Katherine A. Maki Translational Biobehavioral and Health Promotion Branch, National Institutes of Health Clinical Center, Bethesda, MD, USA

Julia McCarthy New York Health Foundation, New York, NY, USA

Ashwini Rajasekaran Centre for Heart Lung Innovation, University of British Columbia and St. Paul's Hospital, Vancouver, BC, Canada

Joan Sabaté Loma Linda University School of Public Health, Loma Linda, CA, USA

Norman J. Temple Centre for Science, Athabasca University, Athabasca, AB, Canada

Methods in Nutrition Research

1

David R. Jacobs Jr and Norman J. Temple

Abstract

- Many different research designs are available for investigating nutrition-related questions. Each has its strengths and weaknesses.
- Much nutrition-related research is carried out using epidemiological study designs.
- Many epidemiological studies use observational designs, including prospective cohort studies, case-control studies, cross-sectional studies, and population studies.
- Results from randomized controlled trials (RCTs) are usually more reliable for causal inference than those from observational epidemiological studies. However, RCTs often have their own limitations.
- A recent development is the use of systematic reviews and meta-analyses. First, the literature is reviewed according to strict criteria. Findings from the studies are then analyzed in order to make pooled risk estimates. These gain power by increasing sample size. This research strategy has proven to be of great value.
- Much mechanistic research is carried out where researchers study the details of body functioning such as physiology and biochemistry. This can reveal the details of body functioning, but using this information in disease prevention is extremely complex.

D. R. Jacobs Jr
Division of Epidemiology and Community Health, School of Public Health, University of Minnesota, Minneapolis, MN, USA
e-mail: jacob004@umn.edu

N. J. Temple (✉)
Centre for Science, Athabasca University, Athabasca, AB, Canada
e-mail: normant@athabascau.ca

N. J. Temple, T. Wilson (eds.), *Pocket Primer for Nutritional Health*,
https://doi.org/10.1007/978-3-032-25402-3_1

- Experiments on animals are often used for nutrition-related research. However, animal models have many differences from the human situation.
- There is evidence of conflict of interest in studies that potentially affect profit of the research funder, most typically in industry funding. This indicates a need for particular care in interpreting such studies.

Introduction

Excellent research designs are essential for efficiently and accurately answering nutrition-related questions. The information generated serves various purposes, including advice from the perspective of health about what foods people should eat, what the food industry should supply, and whether some compounds should be consumed as dietary supplements. Areas of inquiry cover a broad range and include studying molecular mechanisms in cells, animals, and humans; examining what population groups eat; discovering the effects of food, nutrients, and other substances on clinical outcomes and intermediate variables; and investigating how behaviors, policies, and food cost influence food choices.

Over the years many apparent discoveries in various fields of science have been reported in scholarly journals, with seemingly strong supporting evidence, only to be disproved by later research. Nutrition is no exception. Indeed, this problem seems to be especially common in the area of nutrition in relation to diet and health. However, disproved research and rescinded health messages often lead to confusion among the general public.

Knowledge about methodologies used in nutrition research confers a greater ability to comprehend research studies and to critically evaluate new research findings. That is our primary objective in this chapter. Accordingly, we present an overview of the major methods used in nutrition research and describe the strengths and weaknesses of each one. Nutrition is connected to many areas of biomedical science. For that reason, the methods described here are also valid for diverse fields of health. However, this chapter is far from comprehensive. There are excellent articles available that cover this subject in greater detail [e.g., references 1–3].

Fundamental Principles of Research Design

The most common goal of nutrition research is to ascertain the effect of consumption of a food or a substance isolated from food. The outcome variable is often a health construct, including death, disability, a clinical disorder, worsening of a clinical disorder, subclinical disease (such as asymptomatic atherosclerosis), or an intermediate marker variable (assumed to be on the pathway to disease, such as obesity, elevated blood cholesterol, or poor immune status). Alternatively, the outcome variable may be maintenance of health or good quality of life. The research target may be other topics of interest such as cost or the impact of advertising or dietary guidelines on food choices.

Many research studies involve estimating a person's food intake. This is commonly an important source of error [4]. One reason for this is that an individual's food intake varies widely from day to day. Another reason is that people often provide inaccurate answers when questioned on their typical food intake. Fortunately, the inaccuracy of an estimate of dietary intake is typically not great. However, the stated amounts may be correct on average for the population but much too low or high for any given individual.

Another important source of error is confounding. This is defined as the correlation of the exposure and the outcome with other variables. Such correlation may mask true associations between the diet variable and the outcome or produce false associations. For example, in a general population study, whole grain food intake could be positively associated with mortality if whole grain food intake increased sharply with age because age is almost always strongly associated with mortality. Confounding assumes that the correlated variable is not on a causal pathway linking the exposure and the outcome. A similar situation is mediation. Here the correlated variable is on the causal pathway between the intake and the outcome. For example, whole grain food intake may lead to both lower body mass index (BMI) and less incident type 2 diabetes. Here we might conclude that whole grain food intake is associated with diabetes in part because it lowers body weight.

Epidemiological Studies

Epidemiology is the study of the incidence, distribution, control, and prevention of disease. Many epidemiological studies share a common objective: to discover the factors that cause or prevent disease. Epidemiology is central to much nutrition research. Studies in this area aim to describe food or nutrient intake in general or across population subgroups or to understand factors that lead to intake of a given food.

We shall now look at the major types of epidemiological studies. These are often referred to as "observational" as they are based on observing relationships. Another type of epidemiologic study uses experimental testing under a high level of experimenter control. These studies include randomized controlled trials (RCTs) and are discussed later in the chapter.

Cohort Studies

Cohort studies—also known as prospective or longitudinal studies—can potentially yield reliable inferences about causal pathways. The first step in a study is the recruitment of a large number of subjects; typically in the range 30,000–100,000, but sometimes as many as half a million. Cohorts of a small number of people are also useful. There are variations in the inclusion/exclusion criteria: participants may be recruited from the general population; they may be free of serious disease or may be specifically selected because they have a disease (e.g., survivors of childhood cancer).

At baseline the participants are questioned or examined to determine each person's exposure to the particular factors under study, as well as many other variables that might be of importance as confounders, mediators, or effect modifiers. The subjects are then monitored for a long period of time, typically from 5 to 20 years, by which time a sufficient number have developed the conditions or diseases of interest.

After the follow-up period, the data are analyzed to determine the association between dietary and other lifestyle variables and risk of disease. If the participants are known to be free of the disease at study baseline, predictors of incident disease are of particular interest as it is then known that the exposure and outcome occurred in a temporal sequence.

The outcome results for low vs. high intake are presented as risk difference (appropriate for computing attributable risk) or relative risk (RR, appropriate for characterizing disease that develops at a faster rate over time in one group than in another), hazard ratio (HR, used in life table-based methods), or odds ratio (OR, appropriate to methods such as logistic regression that are based on odds [probability of having an event relative to not having it] rather than probability itself).

In long-term studies of an outcome relative to a dietary pattern, a food, or a nutrient, the subjects are typically divided into five equal-sized groups (quintiles) based on their exposure to the variable of interest. However, it may be more appropriate to divide the subjects into fewer groups. It may sometimes be more informative to categorize the subjects into groupings in order to capture important contrasts in level of exposure. Another approach is to examine the association continuously.

The relative risk of the disease in the category with the lowest exposure may be arbitrarily called 1.0. The risk in the other categories is then calculated relative to this reference group. If subjects in the quintile with the highest exposure have a 57% higher risk of the disease, then the RR is stated as 1.57. If subjects in that quintile have a 20% lower risk of the disease, then the RR is stated as 0.80. Typical findings from a cohort study on lifestyle and risk of stroke might be that exercise has an RR of 0.80 while smoking has an RR of 1.9. RR values are normally given for all quintiles, not just the extreme quintiles. The pattern of absolute risks or of RR values is also examined for linearity and thresholds.

The outstanding strength of cohort studies is that information is collected before the disease develops. The next section discusses case-control studies. These are prone to particular sources of error that are avoided in cohort studies. However, cohort studies do have significant sources of error. First, diet assessment may be inaccurate. Another problem is that diet and other aspects of lifestyle, such as smoking and exercise, tend to change over time. It is remarkable, therefore, that in many studies a single assessment in mid-life of smoking, serum cholesterol, and blood pressure predicted heart disease incidence far into the future. But for many variables, data recorded at the start of a cohort study may not reflect actual lifestyle a decade later. For that reason, a single measurement cannot be relied on to predict disease over the long term. Some cohort studies endeavor to minimize this source of error by repeating the data collection every few years.

Confounding was briefly discussed above. It is the greatest challenge in analyzing data from cohort studies. Here is another example. Let us suppose that the findings from a cohort studies reveal that persons with a relatively high intake of dietary factor A have a 50% increased risk of developing disease X. However, further investigation reveals that dietary factor A is associated with smoking which is also associated with disease X. This means that the association between dietary factor A and disease X may be spurious.

Confounding is of great importance in epidemiological studies as lifestyle factors tend to cluster together. Most often this takes the form of some people leading a healthy lifestyle with respect to diet, smoking, and exercise, while others lead a generally unhealthy lifestyle. Another factor associated with a healthy lifestyle is having a higher socioeconomic status. This is most often measured in terms of years of education.

Epidemiologists attempt to overcome the error caused by confounding by making statistical corrections. Let us suppose that a cohort study indicates that red meat has a positive association with risk of colon cancer. The OR is 1.40 when comparing persons in the top quintile for intake of red meat and those in the lowest quintile (i.e., they had a 40% higher risk of developing colon cancer during the period of the study). However, persons with a high intake of red meat typically have a relatively unhealthy lifestyle, such as a lower intake of fruit and vegetables. When the data are corrected for the various sources of confounding, then the OR may be reduced (e.g., to 1.30). This is known as attenuation.

Case-Control Studies

Case-control studies have the same goal as cohort studies, namely to help explain why particular individuals within a population suffer from certain diseases. In case-control studies, a direct comparison is made between healthy subjects and people who already have the disease of interest. Ideally, controls should be selected from the same source population as the cases but this can be difficult to actuate.

This study design is especially appropriate when investigating uncommon cancers and rare diseases. Typically, between 50 and 500 people with the disease of interest are recruited. One (sometimes two or more) healthy—but otherwise similar—person is also recruited for comparison with each case. Subjects are asked about their diet at some past time. By comparing the diet exposure of the two groups, the researchers can estimate the extent to which the diet variable is associated with the risk of the disease (the odds ratio).

Unfortunately, case-control studies can have serious inherent errors [5]. The first is known as "the healthy volunteer effect". When patients with cancer are asked to participate, typically a high proportion agrees. But recruitment of "matched" controls is usually more problematic as a much lower proportion of healthy subjects agree to participate. Moreover, the healthy subjects tend to include an overrepresentation of health-conscious people. The effect of this is that even if patients with a particular type of cancer have a history of eating, on average, an identical diet to the rest of the population, the results of case-control studies will likely indicate that their past diet was relatively unhealthy, such as having a low content of fruits and vegetables. The second problem is recall bias. This refers to the tendency of patients who have recently been diagnosed with cancer to have a distorted recollection of their past diet, usually in the direction of overstating its unhealthy features.

Studies of the relationship between consumption of fruits and vegetables and risk of cancer demonstrate the systematic bias that can be generated by case-control studies. Well over 200 case-control studies have been published and these consistently indicate that a generous intake of fruits and vegetables is strongly protective against several types of cancer. However, findings from large cohort studies, mostly published after 2000, have reported only small protective benefits. As cohort studies are at much lesser risk of systematic bias than are case-control studies, the findings from those studies are much more credible.

Despite these inherent problems, case-control studies still have much value, assuming, of course, that the study was well designed. Exposures that are easy to recall accurately, such as smoking or alcohol consumption, may generate reliable results. Furthermore, if the risk following exposure is short term, such as triggers of sudden death, a cohort study will fail to detect the risk while a case-control study would likely find such risk.

Cross-Sectional Studies

In the cross-sectional design the findings present a snapshot in time. The sample may be selected at random from the general population, either the whole population or a particular group. Cross-sectional studies are often used to look at body parameters that increase by increments, such as BMI and blood pressure. Let us suppose that an investigator wishes to study the relationship between lifestyle and BMI in children. She then recruits several hundred children from the general population and measures both lifestyle factors and BMI. The results might reveal, for example, a positive association between hours of TV watching and BMI.

The information gathered focuses on current lifestyle, including diet, whereas case-control studies usually ask about lifestyle at a former time, before diagnosis of the disease under investigation. Accordingly, cross-sectional studies, for the most part, reveal nothing about temporal sequence whereas case-control studies attempt to determine this. Because of the paucity of information about temporal sequence typical in the cross-sectional design, it cannot distinguish causal direction, even if other aspects of the data lead to a belief that a causal relation is present. Let us look again at the study of the relationship between lifestyle and BMI in children. If that study reveals that children who spend more hours watching TV tend to have a higher BMI, this could mean that TV watching causes children to become overweight, or, conversely, that overweight children tend to watch more TV. Resolving this problem can only be properly addressed by studying children prospectively (i.e., monitoring a cohort of children over several years).

Cross-sectional studies have similar sources of error as those seen with case-control studies.

Population Studies

Population studies—also known as ecological studies—have a long history in epidemiology and have yielded enormous amounts of valuable information. Typically, two dozen or more different countries are compared. Data are collected from each country on food intake and exposure to possible risk factors and these are compared with disease rates. The findings indicate which variables are most strongly associated with each disease. These studies take advantage of the enormous variations around the world in many aspects of lifestyle and disease patterns.

There are several major sources of error in population studies. One is that disease statistics are often unreliable, especially in less developed countries. Food consumption data can also be misleading.

As with other types of epidemiological studies, confounding presents a serious challenge. In the case of population studies, confounding is a reflection of different populations having many lifestyle factors that cluster together. This is best illustrated by studies that have investigated the relationship between diet and chronic diseases of lifestyle. Many such studies have compared populations in highly developed countries and those still living a more traditional lifestyle. What the findings typically reveal is a strong association between a Western diet and many chronic diseases of lifestyle, including colon cancer, coronary heart disease (CHD), and type 2 diabetes. Detailed analysis reveals a strong correlation between all components of the Western diet (such as a high intake of dietary fat, animal protein, and sugar, and a low intake of dietary fiber) and several different diseases. While some of these associations may be a reflection of cause and effect, most are not.

In 1975, Armstrong and Doll [6] published a paper using this methodology in order to explore the relationship between diet and cancer. This paper played a major role in sparking serious interest in the subject. The association between diet and breast cancer mortality in 27 countries illustrates the nature of the findings. The correlations (r) were high for foods of animal origin (approx. 0.75–0.80). The strongest correlation was seen for total fat: 0.89. Conversely, cereals manifested a correlation of −0.70. Many investigators seized on the impressive association between fat intake and breast cancer and became convinced that there must be at least a small fire amid so much smoke. Alas, the search for solid supporting evidence has been largely futile. With the wisdom of hindsight what these findings really show is that a Western diet (and its associated lifestyle) is strongly *associated* with risk of breast cancer. Making inferences as to *cause-and-effect* relationships for single dietary components should only be done with much caution, particularly when the evidence is based solely on ecologic data.

Population studies can be done within a country; for example, comparisons of the states of the United States. The degree of variation between states is obviously far less than that seen between highly developed and developing countries. This has the advantage of greatly reducing the problem of confounding (e.g., differences in disease rates between states are not likely to be due to such factors as dietary intake of meat or sugar or errors in disease diagnosis). However, the relatively small state-to-state variation in nutritional factors and disease rates limits the potential use of this technique. This approach has proven useful in situations of strong geographical variation in dietary status. One recent example of this is using regional variation in sunshine exposure as a surrogate marker for vitamin D status. Results from such studies have lent support to the view that vitamin D is protective against cancer, a topic discussed in Chap. 6.

Population studies have much value. They can be done fairly quickly and usually at low cost. They provide suggestive evidence regarding which aspects of diet and lifestyle affect risk of disease. However, because these studies are prone to serious error, their real value lies in providing suggestive evidence that can then be explored using other, more reliable, methodologies.

Randomized Controlled Trials

Randomized controlled trials (RCTs) have the following key features:

- Subjects are recruited who meet predetermined criteria, such as age, gender, willingness to accept and comply with either intervention or control, and medical history.
- The subjects are randomized into at least two groups: a control group (i.e., untreated, usual care, placebo, or standard treatment) and one or more intervention groups.
- The number of subjects needed is calculated so that the results will be meaningful.
- When possible, studies are carried out "double-blind". This means that neither the subjects nor the personnel who are in direct contact with them know which group each subject is in. This prevents various types of bias.

Comparisons of RCTs and cohort studies are provided in the next section.

Comparative Strengths and Weaknesses of Randomized Controlled Trials Versus Cohort Studies

A key feature of RCTs is that the subjects are randomized into intervention and control groups. As a result there is a high probability that each variable is equally distributed between the groups. This has the great advantage of eliminating the problem of confounding that is so problematic in observational studies. Because of this feature there is a widespread view among medical researchers that RCTs are the "gold standard" and can potentially demonstrate cause and effect. That is generally true for many types of study such as the effectiveness of drugs. Cohort studies, by contrast, are generally viewed as being less reliable. Nevertheless, all study designs have strengths and weaknesses.

Other design criteria also differ between the two research methods. The exposure period in RCTs tends to be relatively short (weeks or a few years), while in cohort studies it is much longer (usually many years). In contrast to RCTs, residual confounding is always possible in cohort studies and other types of observational studies. The possibility of an important biasing effect of residual confounding is reduced when many observational studies in many settings concur, and when they also concur with animal or mechanistic evidence.

RCTs that have been designed to investigate whether a dietary supplement prevents a disease will often use subjects who have a history of the disease or are at high risk of it. For example, a study on cancer prevention may use subjects who have been smokers for many years, while an RCT on whether fish oil prevents heart disease mostly use subjects who have a history of cardiac disease. In each case, the study period may be no more than 3 or 4 years. These design features much reduce the number of subjects needed and therefore the cost of the study. What these RCTs are really studying is whether a dietary change can block the late stages of the disease process. It is unsafe to extrapolate the results to the question of whether the dietary change can achieve primary prevention. By contrast, cohort studies usually recruit only subjects who are reasonably healthy. In many cohort studies, the subjects are then followed up for 10 years or longer. This time period is sufficiently long that it will probably cover most of the stages of disease development from start to finish. With this study design, therefore, the findings tell us whether the dietary change truly prevents the disease. In this respect, cohort studies have the advantage over RCTs.

But what is still uncertain is which method is more reliable in the area of research in the area of diet, health, and disease. A recent study attempted to shine light on this question [7]. A comparison was made of the findings from 97 pairs of studies where diet-disease outcomes had been investigated using both RCTs and cohort studies. The authors came to the conclusion that RCTs and cohort studies have a fairly good degree of agreement. These findings were confirmed in a follow-up study [8].

Systematic Reviews and Meta-Analyses

Research methods are constantly evolving and being improved. An excellent example of this is the move towards systematic reviews and meta-analyses. In many fields of health-related research, a dozen or more human studies are carried out on the same topic. In the traditional literature review, experts have examined each study, one at the time, and made an overall evaluation. A typical conclusion might be: "While the evidence lacks consistency, the majority of studies indicate that a diet with a high content of vitamin X is associated with a reduced risk of disease Y. On balance, this suggests that supplements of vitamin X may reduce risk by 20–30%." This approach has a strong element of value judgment which makes it easy for the reviewer to reach a somewhat biased conclusion.

A trend in recent years has been the publication of systematic reviews and meta-analyses. In a systematic review, the literature is reviewed using search engines according to strict criteria. These criteria might include the date of publication, language, the subject under study, and the type of study. Each paper that meets the criteria is then carefully read and relevant information extracted. The findings from these papers are compiled and then summarized.

A meta-analysis takes this process one step further. Instead of guesstimating a "batting average" of what the results indicate, the reviewers make formal pooled risk estimates. As part of this, larger studies usually receive more weight than smaller ones. Compared with single studies, this research strategy generates results that gain power by increasing sample size.

Mechanistic Research

For many decades, nutritionists have followed the strategy that the road to understanding nutrition is to learn the details of body physiology and biochemistry, such as intermediary metabolism, and thence how the various chemicals in food are involved in health or disease. Certainly, this strategy has revealed a great deal about the role played in the body by many substances found in food. For example, studies of the metabolic actions of vitamins, minerals, and amino acids have revealed why deficiencies of them lead to specific symptoms. It is also true that the discovery of various drugs has grown out of an understanding of metabolic processes and cell physiology, such as cell receptors.

But when we look at the wider arena of health research, this mechanistic strategy has serious weaknesses, as has been argued previously [9]. In particular, in the field of nutrition, the strategy is achieving less and less success in recent decades. The reason for this is really quite simple: the human body is so complex that it is extraordinarily difficult to fully comprehend the finer details of the pathways that lead to health and disease. Compounding this, foods have such great complexity that there are vast numbers of possible interactions between food components and body processes. As a result, attempts to translate an understanding of intermediary metabolism and cellular function into practical nutritional advice on preventing or treating disease seldom achieve success. This argument perfectly complements the parallel arguments we present in our chapter on food synergy (Chap. 8).

Experiments Using Animals

Experiments on animals are comparable to RCTs on humans. In particular, the experimenter sets up different treatment options. Compared to RCTs, experiments on animals have obvious advantages and disadvantages. The advantages are as follows:

- The conditions can be far more rigidly controlled. So if, for example, the investigator wishes to test the effect of a low-fat diet, he can be confident that all the experimental animals have consumed the intended diet, and that there are no other differences between the test and control groups. Such control is rarely possible in studies using human "guinea pigs".
- The animals used in experiments are usually from a single breed and therefore have far less genetic variation than is the case with human subjects.

- Experimental animals can be subjected to hazardous treatments; later they can be killed and their tissues studied. But with humans, needless to say, none of this is allowed.

Experiments on animals do, however, have major disadvantages. This is especially the case in the area of nutrition in relation to health and disease. The dominant problem here is the vast genetic, metabolic, and physiologic gap separating animals from humans. On top of that, humans live a completely different lifestyle to animals in a laboratory. For these reasons, we often find that experimental animals respond very differently from humans when their diets are altered. Animals rarely get diseases of interest for humans, and disease models that exist are only approximations of human disease. For example, some mice have been bred to become obese and to develop diabetes, and in some models, diabetes is induced by a chemical that greatly damages the pancreas. It is uncertain whether these forms of diabetes are relevant to the types of diabetes encountered in humans. Accordingly, while animal models can elucidate biological pathways, findings generated from these studies can only be extrapolated to humans with much caution.

Evaluating the Evidence

Reports regularly appear suggesting that a particular food, nutrient, or other substance in food either increases or reduces risk of a particular disease. Unfortunately, there have been numerous instances of such claims being widely accepted even when the supporting evidence is weak or inconsistent. This inevitably creates confusion before a clearer picture emerges. Well-known examples include the role of dietary fat in various diseases and the possible protective benefit of beta-carotene against cancer.

The process of concluding that an observed relationship is causal can only be made after evaluating all aspects of the evidence. Convergent evidence that comes from different types of research methods, especially RCTs and multiple observational results in which residual confounding is unlikely to be the same across studies, may make causal inference reasonable.

The lesson from how various types of study have led to our present knowledge, often after several major errors were made, is that nutrition research is inherently uncertain. Mechanistic research consumes a large share of research resources. While it has led to important new drug discoveries, it has a poor track record in the area of advancing our understanding of how nutrition is related to the prevention or treatment of disease. It is observational epidemiology and RCTs that have provided the large majority of our information of practical value regarding the relationship between diet and the risk of different diseases and what dietary changes are best in the treatment of different diseases. But we must constantly bear in mind that observational epidemiology is still prone to throwing up many misleading findings while RCTs also have important limitations.

The Problems of Conflict of Interest in Research

A common problem in the area of research is created by conflict of interest [10]. There is an enormous amount of money tied up in the results of research studies. Reports have appeared suggesting that conflict of interest does occur in nutrition research and can distort the findings of studies. Here are two examples that illustrate this problem. Nutri-Score is a front-of-package food label. As described in Chap. 10, this label design appears to be effective for persuading shoppers to select healthier foods. An investigation reported that studies without food industry financial support were 21 times more likely to report that the label is effective compared to studies that had received industry funding [11]. Many studies have investigated the relationship between unprocessed red meat and risk of cardiovascular disease. Studies carried out without financial support from industry were far more likely to report a direct association than were studies that had received financial support [12]. While we must be cautious before drawing firm conclusions, these findings suggest that the research process has been distorted by industry funding in order to generate industry-friendly results.

Summary

Excellent research designs are essential for efficiently and accurately answering nutrition-related questions. The answers are of great value in allowing policies to be developed and for transmitting reliable advice to the population regarding, for example, what foods people should eat and whether particular substances should be consumed as dietary supplements. Areas of inquiry range from molecular mechanisms in cells, animals, and humans; to descriptions of what population groups eat; to effects of food and nutrient intake on intermediate variables and clinical outcomes; and to behaviors, policies, and cost structures that influence the diet.

This chapter has reviewed the major methods employed in nutrition-related research. These are summarized in Table 1.1. Observational epidemiology, which includes several different types of study, has been of major importance in generating a large part of our current knowledge. Cohort studies, in particular, have been of enormous value. Randomized controlled trials (RCTs) are widely viewed as being the most reliable method and can potentially demonstrate cause and effect. However, RCTs have important limitations when used for studying diet-disease relationships. It is debatable whether they are more reliable than cohort studies. The most effective strategy overall is to draw conclusions from the combined results of both observational epidemiology and RCTs. In contrast, a critical evaluation indicates that mechanistic studies produce little of any real practical value in the area of nutrition and health.

Table 1.1 Summary of major methods used in nutrition-related research

Type of study	Design	Advantages	Disadvantages
Cohort studies (prospective cohort studies)	Study of subjects free of disease of interest Long follow-up (years)	Reduced risk of bias as subjects questioned on diet and lifestyle before disease develops Long follow-up allows examining relationship of diet etc., during stages of disease development	Expensive. Requires many years to carry out study Study is observational and reveals association. There are sources of error including recall error and confounding Much caution needed before concluding that associations reveal cause-and-effect relationships
Case-control studies	A direct comparison is made between healthy subjects and people who already have the disease of interest	Requires far fewer subjects, takes far less time, and is far cheaper than cohort studies. Valuable for uncommon diseases	Risk of recall bias as cases have the disease of interest. In addition, there may be error in recall of diet and confounding
Cross-sectional studies	Study of subjects selected at random from the general population, either the whole population or a particular group. Often used to look at body parameters that increase by increments, such as BMI and blood pressure	Takes far less time and is far cheaper than cohort studies. Can provide valuable information on diet and lifestyle factors associated with risk factors for disease such as obesity and elevated blood pressure	As observations are a snapshot in time, it is impossible to determine temporal relationships In addition, this design has the same sources of error as case-control studies
Population studies (ecological studies)	Comparison of diet, lifestyle, and exposure to possible risk factors for disease across multiple countries	Can be done fairly quickly and at low cost. Takes advantage of the great variation in diet, lifestyle, and disease rates around the world	Because of the many variables in diet and lifestyle, findings of associations between diet and disease risk are only suggestive
Randomized controlled trials	Subjects are randomized into two or more groups. One or more groups receive an intervention (such as a modified diet or a dietary supplement). A control group is untreated or receives usual care or a placebo. Follow-up is typically several weeks or months, or a few years	Unlike observational studies, the risk of confounding is eliminated. The findings may reveal cause-and-effect associations	Subjects may already have the disease of interest or be at high risk of it. As a result the study may indicate only the effect of the intervention on the late stage of the disease etiology. By contrast, cohort studies usually have a far longer period of follow-up which may be an advantage

(continued)

Table 1.1 (continued)

Type of study	Design	Advantages	Disadvantages
Mechanistic research	Study of detailed working of body, such as biochemistry and physiology	May reveal mechanisms by which disease develops. Has had success in drug development	Because of enormous complexity of human body, this strategy has a poor record of generating findings of practical value
Experiments using animals	Studies of all types using experimental animals	Experiments are allowed that are not possible on humans. Dietary treatments can be rigorously controlled	Because of enormous differences in genetics between humans and animals, the findings may not be relevant to humans

References

1. Brown AW, Aslibekyan S, Bier D, Ferreira da Silva R, Hoover A, Klurfeld DM, et al. Toward more rigorous and informative nutritional epidemiology: The rational space between dismissal and defense of the status quo. Crit Rev Food Sci Nutr. 2023;63:3150–67.
2. Pounis G, editor. Analysis in nutrition research principles of statistical methodology and interpretation of the results. Cambridge: Academic Press; 2018.
3. Weaver CM, Hodges JK. Designing, conducting, and documenting human nutrition plant-derived intervention trials. Front Nutr. 2021;8:782703.
4. Prentice RL. Dietary assessment and the reliability of nutritional epidemiology research reports. J Natl Cancer Inst. 2010;102:583–5.
5. Willett WC. Fruits, vegetables, and cancer prevention: turmoil in the produce section. J Natl Cancer Inst. 2010;102:510–1.
6. Armstrong B, Doll R. Environmental factors and cancer incidence and mortality in different countries, with special reference to dietary practices. Int J Cancer. 1975;15:617–31.
7. Schwingshackl L, Balduzzi S, Beyerbach J, Werner SS, Zahringer J, Nagavci B, et al. Evaluating agreement between bodies of evidence from randomised controlled trials and cohort studies in nutrition research: meta-epidemiological study. BMJ. 2021;374:n1864.
8. Stadelmaier J, Beyerbach J, Roux I, Harms L, Eble J, Nikolakopoulou A, Schwingshackl L. Evaluating agreement between evidence from randomised controlled trials and cohort studies in nutrition: a meta-research replication study. Eur J Epidemiol. 2024;39:363–78.
9. Temple NJ. Research strategies in nutrition in health and disease: The failure of mechanistic research. Front Nutr. 2023;10:1082182.
10. van Tulleken C, Rollins N, Coombes R. Conflicts of interest: moving towards zero tolerance. BMJ. 2024;387:q257.
11. Besancon S, Beran D, Batal M. A study is 21 times more likely to find unfavourable results about the nutrition label Nutri-Score if the authors declare a conflict of interest or the study is funded by the food industry. BMJ Glob Health. 2023;8:e011720.
12. López-Moreno M, Fresán U, Marchena-Giráldez C, Bertotti G, Roldán-Ruiz A. Industry study sponsorship and conflicts of interest on the effect of unprocessed red meat on cardiovascular disease risk: a systematic review of clinical trials. Am J Clin Nutr. 2025;121:1246–57.

Obesity: A Disease of Overnutrition

2

Catherine M. Champagne and George A. Bray

Abstract

- Obesity is an excess of body fat that is a serious worldwide problem and continues to increase in prevalence.
- Obesity results from increased energy intake from food exceeding what is needed for daily energy expenditure over a considerable period of time, with intake of ultraprocessed foods being one of the culprits.
- Obesity is a risk for many diseases and is often called a disease in and of itself.
- Treatments for obesity include diet, exercise, behavioral therapy, medications, and surgery.

Introduction

This chapter highlights two aspects of obesity: first, obesity predicts the development of many diseases; and second, obesity results from ingesting more energy from food calories over an extended period of time than are expended in daily living. We will deal with several questions designed to focus the discussion:

1. How do we define and measure obesity?
2. Who becomes obese?
3. How does obesity develop? OR What causes obesity?
4. Why is obesity called a chronic relapsing disease process?
5. What can we do to prevent obesity?
6. How effective are treatments for obesity?

C. M. Champagne (✉) · G. A. Bray
Pennington Biomedical Research Center, Baton Rouge, LA, USA
e-mail: Catherine.Champagne@pbrc.edu; George.Bray@pbrc.edu

N. J. Temple, T. Wilson (eds.), *Pocket Primer for Nutritional Health*,
https://doi.org/10.1007/978-3-032-25402-3_2

How Do We Define and Measure Obesity?

The WHO considers obesity an excess of body fat. Body fat and its distribution around the body can be measured with considerable accuracy by several methods. One method is to measure body water by bioelectric impedance analysis (BIA), a technique that assesses body water by resistance of current flow and allows calculation of body fat. The most specific method and also the most expensive involves dual-energy X-ray absorptiometry (DXA), magnetic resonance imaging (MRI), and computed tomographic scans (CT) [1].

Body fat increases with body weight, and thus measurement of body weight has become a surrogate for body fat. For children and adolescents, the Centers for Disease Control and Prevention (CDC) have developed charts for determining the appropriate range of weights for a given height.

For adults, the body weight is usually adjusted for height, and currently the most popular surrogate for body fat in adults is the body mass index (BMI). BMI is widely used in studies of obesity in populations and is a useful starting point for evaluating individuals with possible obesity. However, BMI is not a precise measure of body fat but can be a useful indicator of the need for further evaluation of an individual patient. BMI is an insufficient criterion on its own for the diagnosis of "obesity." In the 2013 AHA/ACC/TOS (**American Heart Association/American College of Cardiology/The Obesity Society**) Guidelines for the Management of Overweight and Obesity in Adults, there is an algorithm showing how BMI is used as a starting point in the evaluation of the patient with obesity [2].

In addition to the BMI, which provides a single number for assessing weight status, there is also interest in where fat is located. This is because fat located in some areas of the body carries greater risk for future diseases than fat in other regions. Central adiposity, that is fat located primarily intraabdominally in so-called visceral fat deposits, carries greater risk of disease. By contrast, fat located on the lower extremities may actually be protective. Patterns of central fat are commonly called "apple shaped" and "pear shaped" to refer to whether the fat is mainly visceral (apple shaped) or more distally located (pear shaped). One way to assess fat distribution is with the Waist Circumference divided by Height which may be better than other measures.

In 2013, Thomas et al. [3] suggested a new geometrical index combining height along with waist and hip circumferences. Called the Body Roundness Index (BRI), this relates to total and visceral body fat and may present as a better tool for health status evaluation. Zhang et al. [4] in a national cohort of individuals from the National Health and Nutrition Examination Survey (NHANES) from 1999 to 2018 found a U-shaped association between BRI and all-cause mortality. This provides evidence of the BRI as a noninvasive, easy screening tool to identify high-risk patients. Schweitzer [5] suggested that the BRI may eventually replace BMI, which does not account for variations based on age, sex, race, or ethnicity.

Who Becomes Obese?

The prevalence of obesity varies by ethnicity and from country to country. In 2015, there were an estimated 1.9 billion people globally who were overweight and 609 million who were obese. In 1980, 26.5% of the world's population were overweight and 7% obese. By 2015, this had risen to 39.0% and 12%, respectively [6]. The rising BMI for several sub-groups in the American population began in the years 1960 to 2000. All groups began to gain weight around 1975 and continued in parallel for the next 25 years. Data suggest that a number of ideas about the cause of obesity may be untenable, including genetic changes, changes in exercise patterns, changes in willpower, and lifestyle factors; the suggestion is rather that some factor in the environment, possibly the food supply, changed about 1970 [7] (Fig. 2.1).

What Causes Obesity?

As noted above, obesity is a disease of overnutrition. It develops because an individual consumes more energy from food over an extended period of time than is needed for daily energy expenditure. The increase in body weight is usually gradual, about 0.5 kg/year (Fig. 2.2). Over 1 year, an adult will eat nearly 800,000

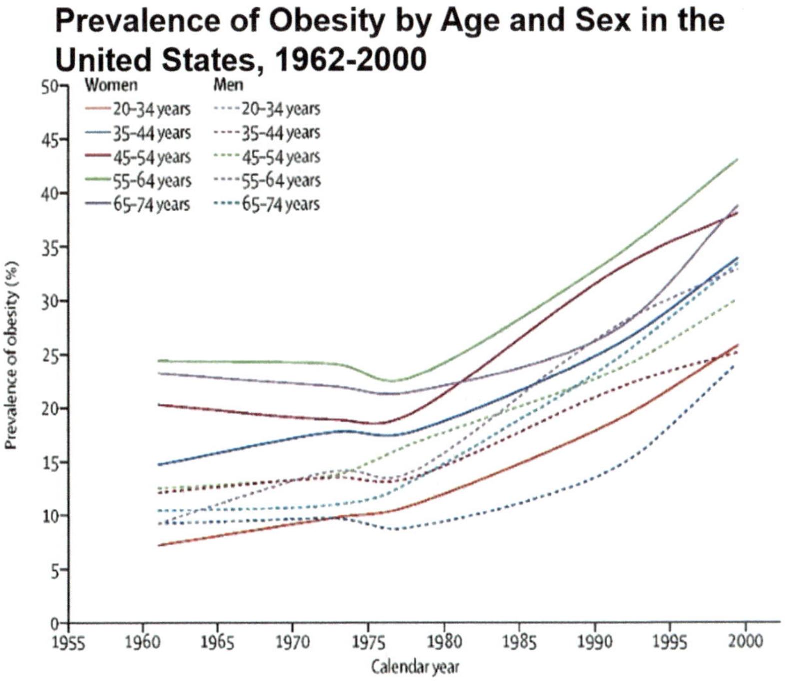

Fig. 2.1 Changes in body mass index among sub-groups of the American Population from 1960 to 2000

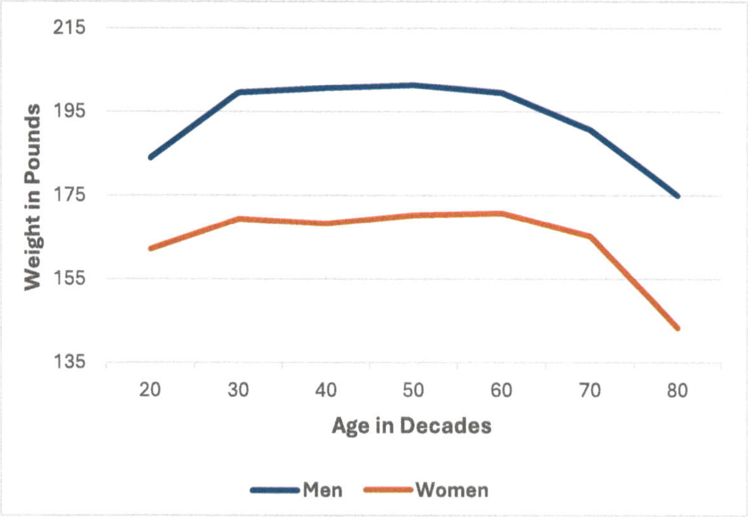

Fig. 2.2 Weight change from age 20 to 80 in men and women [8]

calories. Storage of only 3000 kcal in fat would increase body fat by about 0.5 kg per year.

This imbalance between intake and expenditure is influenced by many factors. People who sleep less are more likely to be obese. People with longer times for consuming food over the day tend to be heavier. Body weight varies with the season, with weight gain in the winter. There is also a sex difference—men tend to be heavier than women (Fig. 2.2). For obesity, the principal lifestyle factors are food and physical inactivity. Other agents include drugs, toxins, viruses, and the microbiome. Age is another important factor: as people grow older, their food intake tends to remain constant while their physical activity declines slowly.

Around the world, tasty, inexpensive, and convenient foods, which are usually high in fat, are abundant and easy to overeat. These foods, often called "ultraprocessed foods," are hard to put down and easily lead to overeating. One suggestion is that a Western Diet, such as is in the United States, has a major impact on disease risk due largely to ultraprocessed food intake. As pointed out by Temple [9], a NOVA system developed in Brazil presented a radically different approach to classifying ultraprocessed foods, further indicating their intake should be reduced. While in somewhat general agreement that ultraprocessed foods are generally high in energy density with high levels of fat, sugar, carbohydrates, and sodium, he suggests that since they encompass a wide range of foods, many are healthy and not obesogenic.

Many aspects of the diet contribute to obesity. Sugary drinks are one. The sugar in soft drinks and fruit drinks is partly "invisible" to the body. Thus, individuals don't "compensate" effectively after drinking them, and they are best avoided [10]. Increasing the intake of healthy foods is associated with more weight loss [11, 12].

Portion sizes have increased, providing more energy to people with each portion, and people tend to eat more when larger portions are provided. The microbiome may also play a role in harvesting energy from foods and thus in obesity [13]. Obesogens, a group of chemical agents used in various products such as plastics, can produce obesity in animals and are of concern. Certain viruses are known to produce obesity in animals, and their potential role in obesity in humans has been suggested in some studies. Some people have genes that in the current "toxic" food environment may become more manifest. The genetic effect can be summarized this way: "Genetic variability loads the gun; environment pulls the trigger; bullets do the damage!" [14].

Several intrauterine events influence postnatal weight and lifetime weight gain [15]. These include maternal smoking and consumption of sugary beverages which should be eliminated during pregnancy. The presence of maternal diabetes can produce large and fat infants at birth.

Our medicated society now produces some medications that cause weight gain. The health professional can use this knowledge to intervene on some occasions by replacing medications that cause weight gain with ones that do not. Table 2.1 is a list of some of these medications and alternative treatments that can be used to avoid weight gain.

Table 2.1 Medications that produce weight gain and possible alternatives

Category	Drugs that may cause weight gain	Possible alternatives
Antipsychotics	Thioridazine; olanzapine; quetiapine; risperidone; haloperidol; perphenazine; clozapine	Molindone Ziprasidone
Antidepressants Tricyclic antidepressants Monoamine oxidase inhibitors Selective serotonin Reuptake inhibitors	Amitriptyline; Nortriptyline Imipramine; Trimipramine Mirtazapine Paroxetine Doxepin	Protriptyline Bupropion Nefazodone Fluoxetine (short-term) Sertraline (<1 year)
Anticonvulsants	Valproate Carbamazepine Gabapentin	Topiramate Lamotrigine Zonisamide
Antidiabetic drugs	Insulin Sulfonylureas Glinides Thiazolidinediones	Acarbose Miglitol Metformin Pramlintide Exenatide; Liraglutide SGLT-2 inhibitors
Antiserotonin	Pizotifen	
Antihistamines	Cyproheptidine	Inhalers Decongestants

(continued)

Table 2.1 (continued)

Category	Drugs that may cause weight gain	Possible alternatives
β-Adrenergic blockers α-Adrenergic blockers	Propranolol Terazosin	ACE inhibitors Calcium channel blockers
Steroids for chronic inflammatory disease	Glucocorticoids	Nonsteroidal anti-inflammatory agents and disease modifying anti-rheumatic drugs
Contraceptives	Progestational steroids	Barrier methods
Endometriosis	Depot leuprolide acetate	Surgical intervention

From: Bray and Champagne [16]

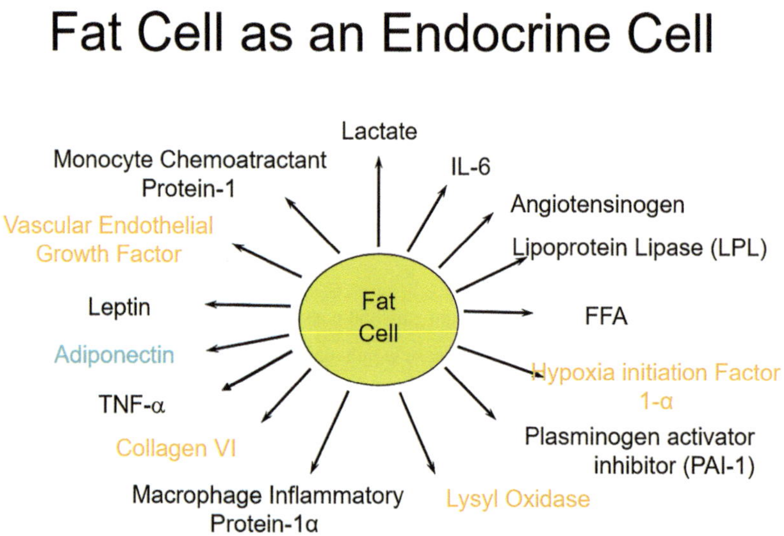

Fig. 2.3 The fat cell is an endocrine cell that produces many secretory products called adipokines. (Source: Bray and Champagne [13]. What is the significance of the different colors?)

Why Is Obesity Called a Chronic Relapsing Disease Process?

Two aspects of body fat help explain the way that obesity damages the body. The first is through the increased weight or mass of fat, which allows obesity to be easily recognized and thus stigmatized. Extra weight can also damage weight-bearing joints. The second way that fat produces disease is through the increased secretion of adipokines by the enlarged fat cells that in turn act on distant organs after traveling through the blood (Fig. 2.3).

Calling obesity a disease goes back centuries. Indeed, Hippocrates, the Father of Modern Medicine in some minds, noted over 2000 years ago that heavier people were at higher risk of dying. For much of the twentieth century, the argument about

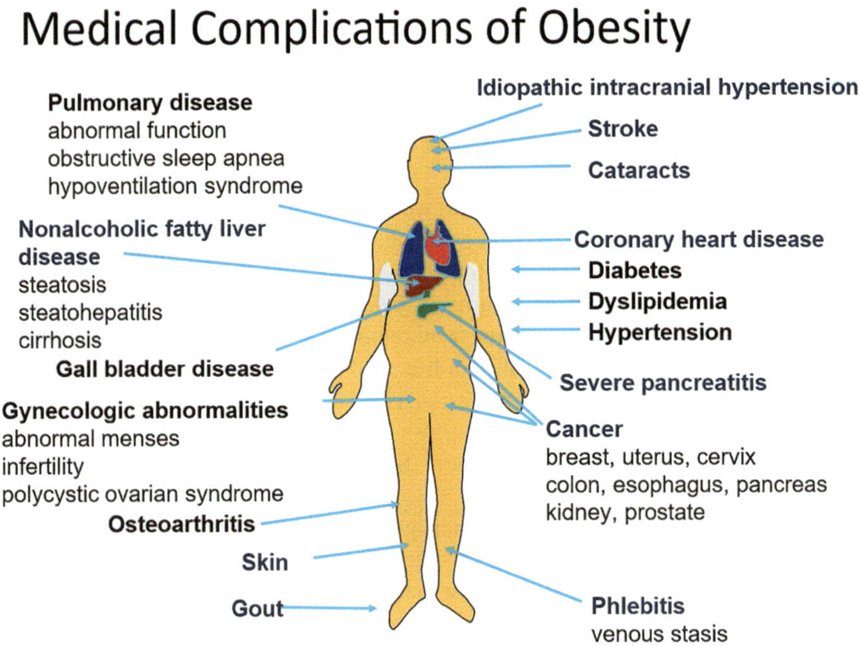

Fig. 2.4 Medical complications associated with obesity. (Source: Bray and Champagne [13])

whether obesity should be called a disease or simply a "condition" has gone on and on. Finally, in 2013, the American Medical Association voted to call obesity a disease. World Obesity, an association of national obesity societies carrying out research in obesity, also called obesity a chronic relapsing stigmatized disease process [17]. The American Association of Clinical Endocrinology echoed this by calling it an adiposity-based chronic disease (ABCD) which focuses attention on the important role that adipokines produced in the adipose tissue have on patients with obesity. Obesity causes many diseases, and these are shown graphically in Fig. 2.4.

What Can We Do to Prevent Obesity?

Findings from epidemiological investigations on obesity indicate that pregnancy, early childhood, and young adulthood represent key periods to intervene and hopefully ward off future weight gain. Pre-pregnant weight and weight gain during pregnancy increase the likelihood of early-onset obesity. Early care in educational settings and schools provide multiple opportunities for prevention in these younger age groups.

Studies of children have shown that exercise and nutritional quality can be improved by lifestyle intervention. However, impacting body weight change is more difficult and often not achieved. Reducing the intake of sugar-sweetened beverages and replacing them with drinking water is a potentially useful strategy.

Studies aimed at preventing weight gain in adults as a group and in special subsets of adults have been less consistent—an area where more work is needed.

How Effective Are Treatments for Obesity?

To decide on effectiveness of treatment, we need a criterion for success [18]. How much weight loss is needed to reduce risk and improve health in people with obesity? It is not necessary for patients to achieve an ideal body weight or even a body mass index <30 kg/m^2 to reap significant health benefits. Modest weight loss of 5–10% improves glycemia, blood pressure, blood lipids, the need for some medications, as well as mobility and quality of life.

The message to healthcare professionals is that significant improvements in health can occur with a modest weight loss of 5% or so, while some patients may need a larger weight loss of 10% or more. Significant weight loss may also reduce mortality.

With all treatments for obesity, there is gradual slowing of weight loss, followed by a high frequency of weight regain when treatment is slowed or stopped [12]. There is also considerable variability in the amount of weight lost along with variability in patient satisfaction with their weight loss. The conclusion from these studies is that a well-designed lifestyle program can provide individuals with the tools they need to lose an average of 8% of their weight and for some to lose more than 15%; this is a very satisfactory outcome. At the other end, however, are an equal number of people who receive little or no benefit in terms of weight loss from this intensive therapy.

Diets are tools that are used by many people to lose weight [19]. A key message from comparison of weight loss diets is that all diets work if followed. In one meta-analysis, the Mediterranean Diet and the DASH Diet were significantly better than comparison diets.

Medications can supplement weight loss produced by diet alone [20]. There are several medications approved by the US FDA for treatment of the patient with obesity, and these are summarized in Table 2.2 [21, 22]. The field has changed dramatically by the substantial weight losses produced by the Glucagon-like peptide antagonists which can produce as much weight loss as seen with surgery [23]. Labeling for all drugs recommends stopping at 12–16 weeks if a 4–5% weight loss has not been achieved.

Surgical treatment of obesity produces the largest weight loss and best maintenance of weight loss of any currently available treatment. There are four main operations in current use: sleeve gastrectomy, Roux-en-Y gastric bypass, laparoscopically placed band or LAPBAND, and the biliary pancreatic diversion. In the Longitudinal Study of Bariatric Surgery (LABS), the median weight loss of 1513 patients who underwent a Roux-en-Y gastric bypass (RYGB) and were followed for 3 years was 31.5% (IQR: 24.6–38.4%); in the 509 patients who underwent laparoscopic adjustable gastric banding (LAGB), weight loss was about half as much or 16.0% (IQR: 8.1–23.1%) [24]. Bariatric surgery can also produce other health benefits including

Table 2.2 Drugs approved for treating obesity in the United States

Name	Trade name	Mechanism of action	Mean weight loss (%) (Mos)
Orlistat	Xenical	Intestinal lipase inhibitor	10.2% 12 months
Phentermine	Many trade names	Sympathomimetic Inhibitor	6.1% 6 months
Phentermine-Topiramate	Qsymia	Sympathomimetic Inhibitor plus GABA blockade	10.9% 12 months
Naltrexone-bupropion	Contrave	POMC neuron stimulation	6.1% 12 months
Liraglutide	Victosa—T2D Saxenda—Ob	GLP-1 receptor agonist	8.0% 12 months
Semaglutide	Ozempic or Rebelsus Wegovy—Ob	GLP-1 receptor agonist	14.9% 16 months
Tirzepatide	Mounjaro—T2D Zepbound—Ob	GIP + GLP-1 receptor agonist	20.9% 17 months
Cagrilintide/Semaglutide	CagriSema—T2D & Ob	GLP-1 Receptor agonist	15–17% 20 weeks
Retatrutide	No official brand name	Triple agonist (GLP-1, GIP, and glucagon receptors	24.2% 48 weeks
Orforglipron	Foundayo—Ob	Small-molecule GLP-1 receptor agonist	9.4–14.7% 36 weeks
Danuglipron	No official brand name	Small-molecule GLP-1 receptor agonist	8–13% 32 weeks

Adapted from Gudzune and Kushner [21] and Ahmed et al. [22]

a significantly reduced risk for developing diabetes, reduced likelihood of myocardial infarction, lower cancer risk in women, and lower all-cause mortality.

Summary

Obesity is defined as an increase in body fat but is usually estimated from measures of height and weight such as the body mass index—Weight (kg)/[Height (m)^2]. But the Rody Roundness Index (BRI) may be a better choice than the BMI in the future. Obesity develops over time, as food intake exceeds energy expenditure due to either ingestion of more food or decreased energy expenditure. Obesity is labeled a chronic disease process because it tends to recur after efforts to lose weight. Obesity is associated with a number of health problems, including diabetes, liver and gallbladder disease, chronic kidney disease, heart disease, and increased risk of mortality. Treatment of obesity can involve use of diets, exercise, behavioral strategies, medications, and surgery. The magnitude of response varies with each of these therapies, and there is substantial variation in the response of individuals to each of these treatments. The challenge of obesity as a nutritional disease is still far from being solved.

References

1. Orsso CE, Silva MIB, Gonzalez MC, Rubin DA, Heymsfield SB, Prado CM, et al. Assessment of body composition in pediatric overweight and obesity: a systematic review of the reliability and validity of common techniques. Obes Rev. 2020;21:e13041.
2. Jensen MD, Ryan DH, Donato KA, et al. Guidelines (2013) for managing overweight and obesity in adults. Obesity. 2014;22(S2):S1–S410.
3. Thomas DM, Bredlau C, Bosy-Westphal A, Mueller M, Shen W, Gallagher D, et al. Relationships between body roundness with body fat and visceral adipose tissue emerging from a new geometrical model. Obesity (Silver Spring). 2013;21:2264–71.
4. Zhang X, Ma N, Lin Q, Chen K, Zheng F, Wu J, et al. Body roundness index and all-cause mortality among US adults. JAMA Netw Open. 2024;7:e2415051.
5. Schweitzer K. Could the body roundness index one day replace the BMI? JAMA. 2024;4
6. Chooi YC, Ding C, Magkos F. The epidemiology of obesity. Metabolism. 2019;92:6–10.
7. Rodgers A, Woodward A, Swinburn B, Dietz WH. Prevalence trends tell US what did not precipitate the US obesity epidemic. Lancet Public Health. 2018;3:e162–3.
8. Fryar CD, Gu Q, Ogden CL. Anthropometric reference data for children and adults: United States, 2007–2010. National Center for Health Statistics. Vital Health Stat. 2012, 11(252)
9. Temple NJ. Making sense of the relationship between ultra-processed foods, obesity, and other chronic diseases. Nutrients. 2024;26(16):4039.
10. Sanmiguel C, Gupta A, Mayer EA. Gut microbiome and obesity: a plausible explanation for obesity. Curr Obes Rep. 2015;4:250–61.
11. Bray GA. From farm to fat cell: why aren't we all fat? Metabolism. 2015;64:349–53.
12. LifeCycle Project-Maternal Obesity and Childhood Outcomes Study Group, Voerman E, Santos S, Inskip H, Amiano P, Barros H, Charles MA, et al. Association of gestational weight gain with adverse maternal and infant outcomes. JAMA. 2019;321:1702–15.
13. Bray GA, Champagne CM. Obesity: understanding and achieving a healthy weight. In: Wilson T, Temple NJ, Bray GA, editors. Nutrition guide for physicians and health care professionals. 3rd ed. New York: Springer; 2022. p. 85–107.
14. Bray GA, Popkin BM. Dietary sugar and body weight: have we reached a crisis in the epidemic of obesity and diabetes? Health be damned! Pour on the sugar. Diabetes Care. 2014;37:950–6.
15. Jacobs DR Jr, Sluik D, Rokling-Andersen MH, Anderssen SA, Drevon CA. Association of 1-y changes in diet pattern with cardiovascular disease risk factors and adipokines: results from the 1-y randomized Oslo diet and exercise study. Am J Clin Nutr. 2009;89:509–17.
16. Vadiveloo M, Sacks FM, Champagne CM, Bray GA, Mattei J. Greater healthful dietary variety is associated with greater 2-year changes in weight and adiposity in the preventing overweight using novel dietary strategies (POUNDS lost) trial. J Nutr. 2016;146:1552–9.
17. Bray GA, Kim KK, Wilding JPH. Obesity: a chronic relapsing progressive disease process: a position paper of world obesity. Obes Rev. 2017;18:715–23.
18. Bray GA, Ryan DH. Evidence-based weight loss interventions: individualized treatment options to maximize patient outcomes. Diabetes Obes Metab. 2021;23(Suppl. 1):50–62.
19. Dinu M, Pagliai G, Angelino D, Angelino D, Rosi A, Dall'Asta M, et al. Effects of popular diets on anthropometric and cardiometabolic parameters: an umbrella review of meta-analyses of randomized controlled trials. Adv Nutr. 2020;11:815–33.
20. Dong Z, Xu L, Liu H, Lv Y, Zheng Q, Li L. Comparative efficacy of five long-term weight loss drugs: quantitative information for medication guidelines. Obes Rev. 2017;18:1377–85.
21. Gudzune KA, Kushner RF. Medications for obesity: a review. JAMA. 2024;332:571–84.
22. Ahmed IS, Tapponi SL, Manaa HM, Soltani A, Hussein EH, Parvaresh FA, HussainZ. A narrative review of weight management strategies: from lifestyle interventions to emerging pharmacotherapies. J Obes. 2026;2026(1):e6556057.
23. Jastreboff AM, Kaplan LM, Frías JP, Wu Q, Du Y, Gurbuz S, et al. Retatrutide phase 2 obesity trial investigators. Triple-hormone-receptor agonist retatrutide for obesity – a phase 2 trial. N Engl J Med. 2023;389:514–26.
24. Courcoulas AP, Christian NJ, Belle SH, Berk PD, Flum DR, Garcia L, et al. Weight change and health outcomes at 3 years after bariatric surgery among individuals with severe obesity. JAMA. 2013;310:2416–25.

Coronary Heart Disease, Cardiovascular Disease, and the Role of Diet

3

Norman J. Temple

Abstract

- Diet plays a major role in the causation of coronary heart disease (CHD).
- A high intake of saturated fatty acids (SFA) was for many years believed to play a major role in the causation of CHD. However, evidence that has emerged in recent years strongly suggests that the importance of SFA in CHD has been much exaggerated. However, increasing the intake of polyunsaturated fatty acids (PUFA) while decreasing SFA may reduce the risk.
- Risk of CHD and cardiovascular disease (CVD) may also be reduced by an increased intake of fatty fish and n-3 polyunsaturated fatty acids (n–3 PUFA) present in fatty fish.
- Several components of the diet increase the risk of CHD and CVD including *trans* fats, sugar-sweetened beverages, and an excessive intake of salt.
- Conversely, a generous intake of fruit, vegetables, nuts, and whole grains are associated with a lower risk.
- Risk reduction of CHD and CVD is associated with eating a healthy diet such as the Mediterranean diet or other healthy dietary patterns.
- Other risk factors include obesity and a sedentary lifestyle.

Introduction

Research over several decades demonstrates that major risk factors for coronary heart disease (CHD) are genetic factors, age, smoking, physical inactivity, hypertension, obesity, and type 2 diabetes. An unhealthy pattern of blood lipids (i.e., dyslipidemia) is strongly associated with risk. This is indicated by a relatively high level

N. J. Temple (✉)
Centre for Science, Athabasca University, Athabasca, AB, Canada
e-mail: normant@athabascau.ca

N. J. Temple, T. Wilson (eds.), *Pocket Primer for Nutritional Health*,
https://doi.org/10.1007/978-3-032-25402-3_3

of total cholesterol (TC) and of low-density lipoprotein cholesterol (LDL-C) and a low level of high-density lipoprotein (HDL-C). The strongest indicator of risk is the ratio of TC to HDL-C [1]. An elevated level of triglyceride is also associated with risk.

A large body of evidence strongly supports a major role for diet in the prevention and treatment of CHD. This chapter examines the relationship between various components of the diet and risk of CHD. Early studies focused on the effect of diet on blood lipids, but it is now accepted that diet affects CHD etiology through a variety of mechanisms. These include insulin resistance, blood pressure, endothelial function, inflammation, and thrombosis.

The main theme of this chapter is the relationship between diet and CHD. However, many of the most informative studies have looked at cardiovascular disease (CVD) in general rather than being focused on CHD. CVD includes stroke and some other types of heart disease apart from CHD. Many of these studies are included in this chapter as they add much valuable information. Moreover, those studies are highly relevant as the causes of CVD and CHD have much overlap.

Dietary Fat and Coronary Heart Disease

The Question of the Fat Content of the Diet

The relationship between dietary fat and health has caused endless confusion. In the 1970s, the great majority of experts held the view that the diet commonly eaten in Western countries has an excessive fat content and this plays a major role in CHD and other chronic diseases including obesity. At that time, the fat content of diets was typically 35–42% of energy intake. A common recommendation was that fat intake should be "less than 30%" of energy intake. This was the recommendation made by the American Heart Association during the years 1986 to around 2005 [2]. The food industry responded by marketing many low-fat versions of common foods such as lean meat and skimmed milk.

But new evidence steadily accumulated, especially from cohort studies, revealing that there is little association between the fat content of the diet and risk of CHD and other chronic diseases. It is now clear that the dietary recommendations that were disseminated during the 1980s and 1990s were counter-productive as they deflected the diet choices of millions of people away from a focus on replacing unhealthy foods with healthy food choices [1]. One problem created by the demonization of fat was that fat-rich foods were seen as inherently unhealthy. This ignores the fact that several fat-rich foods are healthy choices, such as nuts, fatty fish, and olive oil.

In response to these new findings, a much more liberal recommendation regarding fat intake was developed in the USA around 2002. This advocates that fat intake should be in the range 20–35% of energy intake [3].

A Focus on the Type of Fat

While the total amount of fat in the diet has little association with risk of CHD, the type of fat certainly does. This is because different fats have very different effects on blood lipid levels and this is the key mechanism that explains how fat affects risk of CHD.

The Different Types of Fat

The great majority of dietary fats are triglycerides. There are important chemical differences between the different types of fatty acids present in triglycerides.

- Saturated fatty acids (SFA) have no double bonds which means they are fully saturated. They mostly have a chain length of 12–18 carbons. Major sources are foods obtained from animals, such as meat and cheese, and tropical oils.
- Monounsaturated fatty acids have one double bond. Oleic acid, which has 18 carbons, is the most common type. Major sources of these fats include red meat, nuts, olive oil, and canola oil.
- Polyunsaturated fatty acids (PUFA) have two or more double bonds. PUFA are of two types, namely n-6 (omega-6) and n-3 (omega-3). The most common n-6 PUFA is linoleic acid which has 18 carbons and two double bonds. Vegetable oils such as corn oil, sunflower oil, and soybean oil are rich sources. In the case of n-3 PUFA, the most common type is alpha-linolenic acid which has 18 carbons and three double bonds. It is found in vegetable oils. Flaxseed oil is a rich source with smaller amounts in soybean oil and canola oil. Various types of seafood are another important source. Here they are often found as long-chain fatty acids with 20 or 22 carbons and 5 or more double bonds. Rich sources include fatty fish such as herring, salmon, mackerel, and sardines.

Saturated Fats and CHD

There are two key sets of observations:

- Many randomized controlled trials (RCTs) carried out over the past 40 years have established that an increased intake of saturated fats (SFA) leads to an increase in the blood levels of TC and LDL-C. Dietary cholesterol also increases TC and LDL-C levels but to a much lesser degree than SFA.
- A large body of evidence shows that an elevated blood level of TC and LDL-C are major risk factors for CHD.

Based on these observations, researchers concluded that the major dietary factor responsible for the causation of CHD is an excess intake of SFA which leads to a high level of TC and LDL-C and from there to atherosclerosis and finally CHD. A high dietary intake of cholesterol may also, to some extent, add to the harmful effect of SFA. This hypothesis was strongly believed for many years.

If this hypothesis is correct, then cohort studies should clearly and consistently demonstrate an association between intake of SFA and risk of CHD. But this has not been the case. Meta-analyses of cohort studies reveal that a relatively high intake of SFA has only a rather weak association with risk of CHD. Comparison of the extreme quintiles indicates a risk ratio [RR] of 1.06 for total CHD (non-significant) [4] and 1.10 for CHD mortality (significant) [5]. Furthermore, several foods and food groups, which are discussed later in the chapter, manifest a stronger association (either negatively or positively) with risk of CHD. These findings strongly suggest that SFA plays a quite minor role in the causation of CHD [1].

The evidence for a significant role of dietary cholesterol in the causation of CHD is even weaker than in the case of SFA. Its main dietary source is eggs, but there is very little evidence that a relatively high intake of this food is associated with risk of CHD [6].

n-6 Polyunsaturated Fats, Monounsaturated Fats, and CHD

MUFA tend to have a neutral effect on the blood levels of TC and LDL-C. Consistent with this, meta-analyses have suggested no association between intake of MUFA and risk of CHD [7].

In contrast to SFA, an increased intake of PUFA induces a decrease in the blood levels of TC and LDL-C [8, 9]. Of particular importance, PUFA does not lower the HDL-C. The net result is a decrease in the ratio of TC to HDL-C. As noted earlier, this ratio is a strong predictor of risk of CHD. These findings strongly suggest that substituting PUFA for SFA will help prevent the disease. Cohort studies have provided supporting evidence that making this dietary change does indeed lead to a significantly reduced risk of CHD [10–12].

Trans-Fatty Acids and CHD

Trans-fatty acids (TFA) are a special type of PUFA. Whereas the double bonds in PUFA are normally in the *cis* configuration, in TFA, they are in the *trans* configuration. TFA are formed from PUFA during hydrogenation. This process is useful for food manufacturers as it makes liquid oils more solid.

With respect to their effect on blood lipids, TFA are the worst of the worst. Like SFA they raise TC and LDL-C levels. But whereas SFA tend to increase HDL-C, TFA lower it. As a result, TFA cause an increase in the ratio of TC to HDL-C. This can be predicted to increase the risk of CHD. Cohort studies have confirmed that there is a strong association between intake of TFA and risk of CHD [4].

In the past, these fats were commonly present in stick margarine (hard margarine made with hydrogenated oils), cakes, pastry products, cookies, chips, and many fast foods. However, after the dangers of TFA became established, serious action was carried out, including the implementation of government policy, with the goal of removing TFA from food.

Fish, n-3 Polyunsaturated Fatty Acids, and Cardiovascular Disease

Many of the studies referred to from this point in the chapter are mainly concerned with CVD. The rationale for including those studies was explained in the Introduction to this chapter.

The relationship between fish consumption and CVD is examined in Chap. 6. Here we summarize the key findings.

Many prospective cohort studies have demonstrated an inverse association between fish consumption and risk of CVD. This benefit extends to both CHD and sudden cardiac death. This association is seen for fatty fish, such as salmon, herring, mackerel, sardines, and pilchards, but not for fish with a low fat content, such as cod, halibut, and hake. These studies indicate that eating two portions of fatty fish per week reduces risk by around 10–15%.

The obvious explanation for this is that the benefit provided by fatty fish is largely accounted for by n-3 PUFA. If that is indeed the case, then we can predict that supplements of fish oil are protective against CVD. This possibility has been tested in several dozen RCTs. The great majority of the subjects in these studies were either at high risk of CVD or had prior CVD. A clear protective benefit has been reported in many of these studies. The strongest benefit was for sudden cardiac death where, on average, a 35% reduction in risk was seen.

Alpha-linolenic acid (ALA) is a n-3 PUFA found in some plant oils. The possible benefit of ALA has been much less researched than is the case with fish oil. A meta-analysis suggests that ALA has little or no benefit in reducing the risk of CVD [13].

The overall picture that emerges from this research is that fatty fish is protective against CVD. For this reason, fatty fish is widely recommended as a part of a healthy diet. People should be advised to eat at least one or two servings per week. However, the optimum intake may be as much as three or four servings per week.

For persons who choose not to eat fatty fish or who only eat small amounts, it makes sense to consume supplements of fish oil. This is especially the case for those who have CVD or are at high risk of the disease.

Meat and CVD

Cohort studies have reported that the intake of both red and processed meat is associated with an increased risk of CVD. Red meat includes beef, pork, and lamb. Examples of processed meat include ham, sausages, bacon, and salami. A meta-analysis concluded that persons in the top quintile of intake of the two types of meat had a 23% higher risk than those in the bottom quintile [14]. However, other investigators have argued that these associations do not represent cause and effect [15].

How should these conflicting findings be interpreted? Caution suggests that people should minimize their intake of red and processed meat. Also, these foods are linked to other diseases including diabetes and colon cancer. Poultry (chicken and turkey) are much healthier choices as they have no association with cardiovascular risk.

Quite apart from the health effects of meat, this family of foods also has a serious impact on the environment. This is because the production of red meat, especially beef, is a major contributor to the production of greenhouse gases while also leading to rainforest degradation. The magnitude of this environmental damage is considerably greater than that seen with other foods [16]. This subject is discussed in greater detail by Berardy and Sabate in Chap. 13.

Carbohydrates and CHD/CVD

Carbohydrate Intake

As mentioned earlier, for many years, people were given dietary advice to reduce their intake of fat or SFA. The inevitable result is that the lost calories were replaced by an increased intake of carbohydrates. But the dietary advice was seriously flawed as it failed to emphasize that some foods rich in carbohydrates are healthy, whereas others are unhealthy. Eventually it was realized that replacing fat or SFA with sugar or refined grains achieves nothing of value in terms of lowering the risk of chronic disease in general or of CHD in particular. We now examine the relationship between different types of carbohydrate-rich foods and risk of CHD/CVD.

Sugar

The research literature includes many studies that provide valuable information on the relationship between sugar and sugar-sweetened beverages (SSB) and risk of CHD/CVD. RCTs have revealed that sugar causes an increase in the blood pressure and the blood level of triglycerides, TC, and LDL-cholesterol [17]. In terms of the relationship between sugar intake and risk of CHD/CVD, the clearest and strongest evidence is seen in relation to SSB. Cohort studies have reported that each additional daily 250 ml serving of SSB is associated with a 17% greater risk of CHD [18]. Similar findings have been reported for death from CVD [19].

Refined Grains

The relationship between refined grains and risk of CHD/CVD has been less studied than is the case with sugar or whole grains. However, findings from cohort studies strongly suggest that intake of refined grains increases the risk of CHD/CVD [18, 20, 21].

Whole Grains

Cohort studies have demonstrated that whole grains are associated with a reduced risk of CHD [22]. It is estimated that a relatively high intake lowers risk by 27%. Similar findings have been seen for the relationship between whole grains and risk of CVD [14]: persons in the highest quintile of intake have an estimated 13% lower risk compared with people in the lowest quintile.

Fruit, Vegetables, Nuts, and CHD/CVD

Cohort studies indicate that nuts have a protective association with risk of CVD [14]. Fruit and vegetables are another group of foods that have a clear protective association with risk of CHD and CVD. This has been reported in multiple cohort studies [23]. A relatively high intake of these foods reportedly reduces risk by 10–20%. In contrast to these findings, the consumption of potatoes has little or no association with the risk of CHD or CVD [24, 25].

Salt and CHD/CVD

Hypertension is a major risk factor for CHD and of other types of CVD such as stroke. The condition is strongly associated with the amount of salt in the diet. It is predictable, therefore, that as the amount of salt/sodium in the diet rises, so does the risk of CVD. Findings from cohort studies confirm that this is indeed the case as demonstrated by the following meta-analysis that included 617,000 people. Risk of CVD was 19% higher in those with a high intake of sodium compared with persons who had a lower intake [26]. RCTs have confirmed this relationship. Cutting the salt content of the diet lowers the risk of CVD in subjects with elevated blood pressure [27].

Processed foods of many different types are the dominant source of dietary salt. Unless a person is diligent and checks food labels, he or she will probably be unaware of the excessive amounts of salt present in a great many foods. In addition to this source of salt, other important hidden sources include foods purchased in restaurants and fast food. A key component of CHD/CVD prevention therefore requires a major reduction in the salt content of processed food. More immediately, education and encouragement are needed so that the general population better understand how to reduce their salt intake.

Alcohol, Tea, Coffee, and CHD/CVD

The relationship between alcohol intake and risk of CHD/CVD has been studied for several decades. Dozens of cohort studies have reported that alcohol consumption in moderation has an inverse association with risk of CHD and of CVD. In other words, abstainers are at a higher risk than are moderate consumers. The lowest risk is seen at an alcohol intake of about one drink per day but possibly less [28].

However, there has been much controversy in the interpretation of this evidence. Most cohort studies make the assumption that abstainers are typical of the general population except that they choose not to consume alcohol. But this assumption is flawed as it ignores the fact that many people quit drinking after they develop a health problem. People with this history are often at increased risk of CHD. As a result, these "sick quitters" may have a higher risk of CHD than is the case with moderate drinkers [29]. If this is actually the case, then alcohol consumption in moderation has no benefit.

It has long been speculated that red wine may be especially beneficial for the prevention of CHD. This has often been referred to as the French Paradox. The explanation was assumed to be the presence of particular phytochemicals, most notably resveratrol. But careful examination of the evidence as a whole indicates that red wine does not live up to the hype [30]. Cohort studies indicate that all types of alcoholic beverages—wine, beer, and spirits—have a similar association with risk of CHD.

There is no dispute that as alcohol intake climbs above 4 drinks/day so does the risk of CVD, especially stroke and heart failure.

In stark contrast to the harmful effects of alcohol and SSB, consumption of tea has a clear protective association with risk of CVD mortality [18]. This is also seen for coffee, though to a lesser extent [19].

Obesity and CHD/CVD

Obesity is strongly associated with elevated risk for CHD and CVD as well as several CHD risk factors including hypertension, insulin resistance, and dyslipidemia [31].

The distribution of body fat is also important when assessing disease risk. A high waist circumference indicates abdominal adiposity. This may have a stronger association with CHD risk than does high BMI [31]. Commonly used cut-points for waist circumference in the USA are >102 cm (40 in) for men and > 85 cm (35 in) for women. Many other countries use lower cut-points: >90–94 cm (35.5–37 in) for men and > 80 cm (31.5 in) for women.

Physical Activity and CHD/CVD

Aerobic exercise is one more aspect of lifestyle where cohort studies have clearly shown a protective association with CHD [32]. Indeed, a sedentary lifestyle is now recognized as a major risk factor. Much of the benefit of physical activity can be explained by its preventive benefits against several other risk factors such as obesity and type 2 diabetes.

Cohort studies have observed that muscle strengthening exercise (weight training) has a protective association with risk of CVD. This association is remarkably strong with reports indicating a risk reduction of 20–25% in comparisons of those who regularly engage in this form of exercise as compared to those who don't [33].

Conclusions

There have been enormous developments over the past half century in our understanding of how the diet affects the risk of CHD. From around 1974, it was widely believed that the dominant dietary factor responsible for the causation of CHD is an excessive intake of saturated fatty acids (SFA). This hypothesis appeared to make good sense as an increase in the intake of SFA causes a rise in the blood level of total cholesterol (TC) which is a major risk factor for CHD. But by about 2014, much evidence had accumulated that cast serious doubt on that hypothesis. In particular, cohort studies failed to demonstrate a clear association between intake of SFA and risk of CHD. Instead, meta-analyses indicate that persons with a relatively high intake of SFA have only a modestly higher risk of CHD (about 5–10% higher) compared with those with a low intake.

An important consideration when looking at the relationship between intake of SFA and risk of CHD is the question of other foods and macronutrients. People who have a low intake of SFA must have a higher amount of other macronutrients in order to replace the lost calories. If the reduced intake of SFA is replaced by carbohydrates in the form of sugar and refined grains, there is little effect on risk of CHD. This can be explained by the fact that replacing dietary SFA with sugar and refined grains lowers the TC, the LDL-C, and the HDL-C. This results in a minimal change in the ratio of TC to HDL-C. It is important to bear in mind that the ratio of TC to HDL-C is a much stronger indicator of risk of CHD than is TC as a single variable. But if SFA is replaced by PUFA, then we find a different outcome, namely a reduced risk of CHD. This is consistent with the fact that replacing dietary SFA with PUFA lowers the LDL-C but without lowering the HDL-C. As a result the ratio of TC to HDL-C is decreased.

Several other components of the diet are strongly associated with risk of CHD/CVD, either positively or negatively. Factors that increase risk include sugar-sweetened beverages (SSBs) and an excessive intake of salt. By contrast, risk may be reduced by an increased intake of fatty fish and the n-3 polyunsaturated fatty acids (n–3 PUFA) present in this fish. Similarly, a generous intake of whole grains, fruit, vegetables, and nuts are associated with a lower risk.

Those foods or components of food that are protective against CHD/CVD are the same ones that are widely recognized as being beneficial for health and protective against a variety of chronic diseases. In summary, a diet that prevents CHD/CVD is a healthy diet. We can flip this around: the dominant cause of CHD/CVD is an unhealthy diet.

The findings discussed in this chapter are of enormous importance and have led to a radical change in the dietary strategy for the prevention of CHD/CVD. There is now a focus on foods, food groups, and dietary patterns. The Mediterranean diet is the diet pattern with the strongest evidence supporting a positive effect on cardiovascular health [34]. The DASH diet also has solid supporting evidence, not only for CHD/CVD but also for hypertension [35]. Over the last few years much attention has turned to the Planetary Health Diet which also has a clear protective association with risk of CHD/CVD [36, 37]. These diets are discussed in detail in Chap. 5.

Table 3.1 Key aspects of the relationship between diet and risk of CHD/CVD

Area of nutrition	Specific dietary component, food, or food pattern	Association with risk of CHD/CVD[a]
Component of foods	Saturated fatty acids (SFA)	↑
	Trans-fatty acids (TFA)	↑↑
	Polyunsaturated fatty acids (PUFA)	↓↓
	Sodium/salt	↑↑
Foods	Sugar-sweetened beverages	↑↑
	Red meat, processed meat	(↑↑?)
	Refined grains	↑↑
	Whole grains	↓↓
	Fruit and vegetables	↓↓
	Fatty fish (and n-3 polyunsaturated fatty acids)	↓↓
	Nuts	↓↓
Dietary patterns	Western diet (typical diet eaten in USA and UK)	↑↑
	Mediterranean diet	↓↓
	DASH diet	↓↓
	Planetary health diet	↓↓

[a]Risk increases/decreases by approximately 5–10% (one arrow) or 10–20% (two arrows)

Table 3.1 presents a summary of the key aspects of the relationship between diet and risk of CHD/CVD.

Finally, we must bear in mind that not only does diet play a major role in the causation and prevention of CHD/CVD but so also do other aspects of lifestyle. Risk of CHD/CVD can be reduced by the avoidance of excess weight gain and engaging in regular exercise, both aerobic exercise and muscle strengthening exercise.

References

1. Temple NJ. Fat, sugar, whole grains and heart disease: 50 years of confusion. Nutrients. 2018;10:39.
2. Krauss RM, Deckelbaum RJ, Ernst N, Fisher E, Howard BV, Knopp RH, et al. Dietary guidelines for healthy American adults. A statement for health professionals from the Nutrition Committee, American Heart Association. Dietary guidelines for healthy American adults. A statement for health professionals from the Nutrition Committee, American Heart Association. Circulation. 1996;94:1795–800.
3. Institute of Medicine. Dietary reference intakes for energy, carbohydrate, fiber, fat, fatty acids, cholesterol, protein, and amino acids. Washington: The National Academies Press; 2005.
4. de Souza RJ, Mente A, Maroleanu A, Cozma AJ, Ha V, Kishibe T, et al. Intake of saturated and trans unsaturated fatty acids and risk of all cause mortality, cardiovascular disease, and type 2 diabetes: systematic review and meta-analysis of observational studies. BMJ. 2015;351:h3978.
5. Mazidi M, Mikhailidis DP, Sattar N, Toth PP, Judd S, Blaha MJ, et al. International lipid expert panel (ILEP) & lipid and blood pressure meta-analysis collaboration (LBPMC) group.

Association of types of dietary fats and all-cause and cause-specific mortality: A prospective cohort study and meta-analysis of prospective studies with 1,164,029 participants. Clin Nutr. 2020;39:3677–86.

6. Drouin-Chartier J, Chen S, Li Y, Schwab AL, Stampfer MJ, Sacks FM, et al. Egg consumption and risk of cardiovascular disease: three large prospective US cohort studies, systematic review, and updated meta-analysis. BMJ. 2020;368:m513.
7. Chowdhury R, Warnakula S, Kunutsor S, Crowe F, Ward HA, Johnson L, et al. Association of dietary, circulation, and supplement fatty acids with coronary risk. Ann Intern Med. 2014;160:398–406.
8. Carson JAS, Lichtenstein AH, Anderson CAM, Appel LJ, Kris-Etherton PM, Meyer KA, et al. Dietary cholesterol and cardiovascular risk: a science advisory from the American Heart Association. Circulation. 2020;141:e39–53.
9. Zhu Y, Bo Y, Liu Y. Dietary total fat, fatty acids intake, and risk of cardiovascular disease: a dose-response meta-analysis of cohort studies. Lipids Health Dis. 2019;18:91.
10. Farvid MS, Ding M, Pan A, Sun Q, Chiuve SE, Steffen LM, et al. Dietary linoleic acid and risk of coronary heart disease: a systematic review and meta-analysis of prospective cohort studies. Circulation. 2014;130:1568–78.
11. Virtanen JK. Randomized trials of replacing saturated fatty acids with n-6 polyunsaturated fatty acids in coronary heart disease prevention: not the gold standard? Prostaglandins Leukot Essent Fat Acids. 2018;133:8–15.
12. Maki KC, Eren F, Cassens ME, Dicklin MR, Davidson MH. ω-6 polyunsaturated fatty acids and cardiometabolic health: current evidence, controversies, and research gaps. Adv Nutr. 2018;9:688–700.
13. Jiang H, Wang L, Wang D, Yan N, Li C, Wu M, et al. Omega-3 polyunsaturated fatty acid biomarkers and risk of type 2 diabetes, cardiovascular disease, cancer, and mortality. Clin Nutr. 2022;41:1798–807.
14. Bhandari B, Liu Z, Lin S, Macniven R, Akombi-Inyang B, Hall J, et al. Long-term consumption of 10 food groups and cardiovascular mortality: a systematic review and dose response meta-analysis of prospective cohort studies. Adv Nutr. 2023;14:55–63.
15. Hill ER, O'Connor LE, Wang Y, Clark CM, McGowan BS, Forman MR, et al. Red and processed meat intakes and cardiovascular disease and type 2 diabetes mellitus: An umbrella systematic review and assessment of causal relations using Bradford Hill's criteria. Crit Rev Food Sci Nutr. 2024;64:2423–40.
16. Jennings R, Henderson AD, Phelps A, Janda KM, van den Berg AE. Five U.S. dietary patterns and their relationship to land use, water use, and greenhouse gas emissions: implications for future food security. Nutrients. 2023;15:215.
17. Te Morenga LA, Howatson AJ, Jones RM, Mann J. Dietary sugars and cardiometabolic risk: systematic review and meta-analyses of randomized controlled trials of the effects on blood pressure and lipids. Am J Clin Nutr. 2014;100:65–79.
18. Bechthold A, Boeing H, Schwedhelm C, Hoffmann G, Knüppel S, Iqbal K, et al. Food groups and risk of coronary heart disease, stroke and heart failure: a systematic review and dose-response meta-analysis of prospective studies. Crit Rev Food Sci Nutr. 2019;59:1071–90.
19. Bhandari B, Zeng L, Grafenauer S, Schutte AE, Xu X. Long-term consumption of 6 different beverages and cardiovascular disease-related mortality: a systematic review and meta-analysis of prospective cohort studies. Curr Dev Nutr. 2024;8:102095.
20. Reynolds A, Mann J, Cummings J, Winter N, Mete E, Te Morenga L. Carbohydrate quality and human health: a series of systematic reviews and meta-analyses. Lancet. 2019;393:434–45.
21. Jones JM, García CG, Braun HJ. Perspective: whole and refined grains and health-evidence supporting "make half your grains whole". Adv Nutr. 2020;11:492–506.
22. Liu H, Zhu J, Gao R, Ding L, Yang Y, Zhao W, et al. Estimating effects of whole grain consumption on type 2 diabetes, colorectal cancer and cardiovascular disease: a burden of proof study. Nutr J. 2024;23:49.

23. Zurbau A, Au-Yeung F, Blanco Mejia S, Khan TA, Vuksan V, Jovanovski E, et al. Relation of different fruit and vegetable sources with incident cardiovascular outcomes: a systematic review and meta-analysis of prospective cohort studies. J Am Heart Assoc. 2020;9:e017728.
24. Schwingshackl L, Schwedhelm C, Hoffmann G, Boeing H. Potatoes and risk of chronic disease: a systematic review and dose-response meta-analysis. Eur J Nutr. 2019;58:2243–51.
25. So J, Avendano EE, Raman G, Johnson EJ. Potato consumption and risk of cardio-metabolic diseases: evidence mapping of observational studies. Syst Rev. 2020;9:274.
26. Wang YJ, Yeh TL, Shih MC, Tu YK, Chien K. Dietary sodium intake and risk of cardiovascular disease: a systematic review and dose-response meta-analysis. Nutrients. 2020;12:2934.
27. Cook NR, He FJ, MacGregor GA, Graudal N. Sodium and health-concordance and controversy. BMJ. 2020;369:m2440.
28. Wood AM, Kaptoge S, Butterworth AS, Willeit P, Warnakula S, Bolton T, et al. Risk thresholds for alcohol consumption: combined analysis of individual-participant data for 599 912 current drinkers in 83 prospective studies. Lancet. 2018;391:1513–23.
29. Fillmore KM, Stockwell T, Chikritzhs T, Bostrom A, Kerr W. Moderate alcohol use and reduced mortality risk: systematic error in prospective studies and new hypotheses. Ann Epidemiol. 2007;17(5 Suppl):S16–23.
30. Haseeb S, Alexander B, Baranchuk A. Wine and cardiovascular health: a comprehensive review. Circulation. 2017;136:1434–48.
31. Piché ME, Poirier P, Lemieux I, Després JP. Overview of epidemiology and contribution of obesity and body fat distribution to cardiovascular disease: an update. Prog Cardiovasc Dis. 2018;61:103–13.
32. Cleven L, Krell-Roesch J, Nigg CR, Woll A. The association between physical activity with incident obesity, coronary heart disease, diabetes and hypertension in adults: a systematic review of longitudinal studies published after 2012. BMC Public Health. 2020;20:726.
33. Giovannucci EL, Rezende LFM, Lee DH. Muscle-strengthening activities and risk of cardiovascular disease, type 2 diabetes, cancer and mortality: a review of prospective cohort studies. J Intern Med. 2021;290:789–805.
34. Rosato V, Temple NJ, La Vecchia C, Castellan G, Tavani A, Guercio V. Mediterranean diet and cardiovascular disease: a systematic review and meta-analysis of observational studies. Eur J Nutr. 2019;58:173–91.
35. Chiavaroli L, Viguiliouk E, Nishi SK, Blanco Mejia S, Rahelić D, Kahleová H, et al. DASH dietary pattern and cardiometabolic outcomes: an umbrella review of systematic reviews and meta-analyses. Nutrients. 2019;11:338.
36. Rockström J, Thilsted SH, Willett WC, Gordon LJ, Herrero M, Hicks CC, et al. The EAT-Lancet Commission on healthy, sustainable, and just food systems. Lancet. 2025;406:1625–700.
37. Liu J, Shen Q, Wang X. Emerging EAT-Lancet planetary health diet is associated with major cardiovascular diseases and all-cause mortality: A global systematic review and meta-analysis. Clin Nutr. 2024;43:167–79.

Ultra-Processed Foods: Their Impact on Health

4

Norman J. Temple

Abstract

- The NOVA System is a classification that divides food into groups based on the extent of processing.
- This classification system is inconsistent with the evidence from nutrition science.
- Ultra-processed foods (UPF) is one group within that system and includes foods that are highly processed and contain various additives.
- Most UPF are unhealthy but others are reasonably healthy.
- Intake of UPF is associated with various chronic diseases of lifestyle. This is probably mainly due to a small number of unhealthy foods such as processed meat and sugar-sweetened beverages.
- Many UPF are hyperpalatable and have a high energy density which may lead to an excessive energy intake and obesity.

What Are Ultra-Processed Foods?

The conventional approach is to classify foods based on their dominant ingredients and composition. Thus, for example, cereals are normally placed together as a single food group. Dietary recommendations are based on advising people to eat a diet based on foods that are strongly associated with a reduced risk of chronic diseases of lifestyle (CDL) [1–4]. The recommended diet also aims to ensure that people consume enough of all macronutrients and micronutrients, especially essential

N. J. Temple (✉)
Centre for Science, Athabasca University, Athabasca, AB, Canada
e-mail: normant@athabascau.ca

N. J. Temple, T. Wilson (eds.), *Pocket Primer for Nutritional Health*,
https://doi.org/10.1007/978-3-032-25402-3_4

nutrients (vitamins, minerals, essential oils, etc.) that the body cannot synthesize, while avoiding an excessive intake of potentially harmful substances and of energy.

Ultra-processed foods (UPF) are one of the food groups in the NOVA System. This is a radically different approach to the classification of foods. The system was developed in Brazil around 2010 by Monteiro and colleagues [5]. The system was later modified [6, 7]. A key feature is that it disregards the nutrient composition of foods. Instead, foods are classified into one of four food groups based on the extent to which the food has been processed and the purpose of the processing. The four food groups are as follows.

1. Unprocessed or minimally processed foods. These include fresh, dry, or frozen fruits or vegetables, grains, legumes, meat, fish, and milk.
2. Processed culinary ingredients including sugar, oils, fats, salt, and other constituents extracted from foods and used in kitchens to make culinary preparations.
3. Processed foods. These include such foods as canned fish and vegetables, simple breads, and cheeses, which are manufactured by only adding salt, sugar, oil, or other processed culinary ingredients to unprocessed or minimally processed foods.
4. Ultra-processed foods (UPF). These are foods that are made from mixtures of ingredients that are the product of industrial processes. UPF contain products extracted from actual foods combined with various additives.

Those who advocate in favor of this system make the bold claim that all UPF are unhealthy. Accordingly, their single most important dietary recommendation is the reduction or elimination of UPF.

Many nutrition experts have declared their support for the NOVA System. For example, Lawrence [8] stated: "UPF is a fit-for-purpose concept for guiding nutrition policy activities to tackle unhealthy and unsustainable diets." Brazil has gone one step further and advised the population to cut its intake of UPF [9].

An Overview of Dietary Recommendations: The Conventional System Versus the NOVA System

As indicated above, conventional approaches to food classification and dietary recommendations are based on the best available evidence coming from studies of the relationship between diet and health. In other words, following the dietary recommendations should lead to enhanced health and a major reduction in risk of CDL. We see this approach in the Dietary Guidelines for Americans [10]. Likewise, we see this in the design of the food guides used in most countries which, today, typically recommend a generous intake of fruit, vegetables, and whole grains. The design of front-of-package food labels also follows this approach. This is exemplified by Nutri-Score [11, 12]. Foods are divided into five groups based on their content of various components. The foods classified as most healthy are those with a low content of saturated fat, sugar, sodium, and energy but a higher content of protein, dietary fiber, fruits, vegetables, pulses, nuts, and healthy oils such as olive and canola [13].

A recent trend in dietary recommendations centers on dietary patterns [14]. This is exemplified by the recommendation that has been made by many nutrition experts that people should eat a Mediterranean diet [15]. Again, the supporting evidence comes from studies that leave little doubt that people who follow this diet are at reduced risk of many forms of CDL.

The NOVA System, as stated earlier, is based on the extent to which a food has been processed. It disregards both the nutritional composition of the food and the available evidence that indicates whether the food increases the risk of different types of CDL or is protective.

Not surprisingly, the NOVA System has been much criticized [16–18]. For example, a food may be a good source of whole grains and should therefore be viewed as likely to be a healthy choice. But if the grain has been processed and it contains several additives, then it will probably be included with UPF. This misleading classification is the case with some types of bread. The mirror image of this problem is seen with red meat. Multiple studies have provided clear evidence that regular consumers of this food have an increased risk of cardiovascular mortality [19] and of several types of cancer [20]. Red meat is commonly eaten as a steak which is clearly not a UPF as it is unprocessed or minimally processed. The NOVA System is therefore placing this unhealthy food in the same group as healthy foods.

Foods with a relatively high content of salt can also be misclassified. The presence of this substance pushes food in the direction of being unhealthy. Let us compare tomato juice with and without added salt. The NOVA System classifies each as a "processed food." We see the same problem with canned fruit. It is also classed as a "processed food" regardless of whether the food contains added sugar.

In each of the above examples—bread containing whole grains, red meat, and various foods with a high content of salt or sugar—the NOVA System is prone to providing misleading information regarding whether a food is healthy or not. We can see the problem more clearly by comparing the NOVA System with Nutri-Score, the front-of-package food labeling system that was discussed above. As this system divides foods into five groups based on the nutritional value of the food, it is a far more reliable source of accurate nutritional guidance.

The serious flaws in the NOVA System were also demonstrated by the following study [21]. The researchers formulated a diet based on foods commonly eaten in the USA. The diet was designed to consist mainly of UPF while also being consistent with the recommendations stated in the Dietary Guidelines for Americans [10]. Despite the fact that 91% of the food energy came from UPF, the diet was still relatively healthy.

The Relationship Between Ultra-Processed Foods and Disease

The NOVA System is based on the premise that UPF are unhealthy and should therefore be eliminated from the diet. If the system works as intended, then epidemiological studies should reveal a clear association between intake of UPF and risk of CDL. Findings, mainly from prospective cohort studies, have indeed demonstrated this. The strongest associations are seen in relation to obesity, cardiovascular disease (CVD), type 2 diabetes, common mental disorders (especially depression), and all-cause mortality [22–24]. Similar associations, albeit less strong, have been reported for cancer and hypertension.

These findings pose the obvious question: why is the intake of UPF associated with an increased risk of CDL in light of the flaws in the NOVA System? Fortunately, there is an obvious explanation for this. Most foods classed as UPF (but not all) are unhealthy. The UPF classification is best viewed as a crude indicator that particular foods are unhealthy [18].

This also helps explain why the findings from cohort studies have a lack of consistency. A major reason for this is that there is much variation in the types of foods classed as UPF. This is because there is no widely accepted definition of the term.

Going one step further, we can predict that if the findings from cohort studies were analyzed in detail, we would discover that for each type of CDL, some types of UPF are associated with the disease while others are not. We can confidently predict that the foods most strongly associated with risk of CDL are those that are classed as unhealthy based on conventional systems for categorizing foods. Indeed, several cohort studies have done that and generated findings that support this viewpoint [18].

Ultra-Processed Foods and Obesity

The evidence presented so far in this chapter is largely negative as regards the value of the NOVA System. Classifying a food as UPF seems little more than a crude indicator that the food is unhealthy. But when we turn our attention to the subject of excess weight gain and obesity, a different picture appears.

The obesity epidemic first appeared in the USA in the late 1970s [25]. It then spread across the Western world, and by the 1990s, it was having an impact on less affluent countries [26]. In a previous paper, I presented the case that the huge growth in intake of UPF provides the best explanation for the epidemic [25].

A common characteristic of UPF is that they are able to bypass the appetite control system. As a result, the consumption of these foods leads to an excessive energy intake. Such foods are best described as being hyperpalatable. Because such large numbers of UPF are hyperpalatable and lead to uncontrolled eating, some researchers have even argued that UPF are addictive and act much like drugs [27].

The types of UPF most likely to have this effect are those that have a high content of both fat and carbohydrates. Dicken et al. [28] made a slightly different argument, namely that the most hyperpalatable types of UPF are those that have a high content of fat, sugar, carbohydrates, and sodium. This composition is a feature of huge numbers of UPF. This was demonstrated in a study carried out in the UK. A large selection of foods were divided into groups based on the NOVA System. A high proportion of UPF met the definition of being hyperpalatable but only a small fraction of minimally processed foods (68.0% vs 13.4%). This strongly suggests that UPF, in general, are hyperpalatable.

Most UPF have a high energy density. This is another major reason why eating UPF induces a high energy intake and is closely linked to obesity. In the above study of foods eaten in the UK, the researchers calculated the energy density of different classes of food. The median energy density of UPF was more than double that of minimally processed food (243 vs 94 kcal per 100 g) [28].

Strong supporting evidence for the role of energy density in leading to a higher energy intake was shown in a systematic review and meta-analysis of 38 randomized controlled trials [29]. In each trial, subjects were fed meals with either a higher or lower median energy density (150 vs 110 kcal per 100 g). When subjects were given meals with a higher energy density, their energy intake was higher by, on average, 223 kcal per day. If this extra energy intake were repeated at a single meal every day and a fraction of it was turned into body fat, it would lead to an increase in the average BMI across the population that can easily explain what caused the obesity epidemic.

Findings from an especially informative randomized controlled trial provided additional evidence for the impact of UPF on energy intake [30]. Two groups of subjects were fed a diet based on either UPF or minimally processed foods. No limits were placed on the amount of food eaten during the 2 weeks of the study. Those eating the UPF diet consumed 508 kcal per day more food energy. Consistent with this, their average weight increased by 0.9 kg.

The evidence presented above demonstrates that UPF, in general, are both hyperpalatable and have a high energy density in comparison with minimally processed foods. This combination exerts a synergistic action on the appetite. Inevitably, therefore, when generous amounts of UPF are included in the diet, most people consume an excessive energy intake. None of this is an accident. The credit belongs to food technologists. They have applied their expertise to the design of UPF with the goal of making them appealing to the eye and enjoyable to eat.

We must be careful not to oversimplify. Nutrition is complex which means that generalizations will always have many exceptions. In particular, two additional comments need to be added. First, as stressed earlier, UPF is an umbrella term and includes many relatively healthy foods. Such foods, for example, bread with a high content of whole grains, are not hyperpalatable. Second, in terms of causing an excess intake of food energy, foods classified as "processed" according to the NOVA scheme are closer to UPF than to minimally processed foods.

The cause of obesity has been intensively investigated for decades. Researchers have looked at many aspects of the diet such as the amount of fat or fiber and portion sizes. The evidence presented here and in a previous paper [25] leads to the conclusion that UPF play a major causal role.

Thousands of different UPF are available. They are sold everywhere, are heavily marketed, and are a relatively cheap source of food energy. It is therefore unjustified to accuse people who seem addicted to UPF and become obese of being guilty of gluttony. Rather, they should be seen as victims of an obesogenic environment.

Ultra-Processed Foods and Nutrition Advice

The information presented in this chapter has important implications for nutrition advice that is delivered to the population. The evidence demonstrates that there are serious weaknesses in the claim that UPF are inherently unhealthy. Moreover, some unhealthy foods, such as steaks, are not included within the UPF group. It follows, therefore, that there is no reason to modify conventional systems for classifying foods and making dietary recommendations. Very little would be gained by incorporating UPF into food guides, front-of-package food labels, and similar documents. Indeed, to do that would add more noise than signal.

We now have strong evidence that UPF play a central role in the causation of obesity. Does this change the above conclusions? The answer is no. Food guides encourage people to eat a diet where most food comes from whole grains, fruit, vegetables, and other healthy foods. A person who follows that advice will automatically eat very little UPF. This will also be the case if consumers select foods based on the information given in well-designed front-of-package food labels, such as Nutri-Score. The conventional systems for making dietary recommendations therefore achieve the best of all worlds: they are solidly based on nutrition science, they strongly encourage people to exclude obesogenic foods (especially obesogenic UPF), while also presenting advice that is clear and avoids confusion.

Conclusion

Table 4.1 summarizes the key points of this chapter. The NOVA System of food classification is radically different from conventional systems. It disregards the nutritional value of foods and whether their intake is associated (positively or negatively) with risk of CDL. UPF is an umbrella term that lumps together foods that are highly processed and contain assorted additives, particularly industrially produced additives.

Most UPF are unhealthy but others are reasonably healthy. Conversely, some unhealthy foods are not classified as UPF. This classification system is clearly inconsistent with the evidence coming from nutrition science. However, the findings from cohort studies reveal that intake of UPF is associated with risk of obesity, CVD, type 2 diabetes, common mental disorders (especially depression), cancer, hypertension, and all-cause mortality. At first glance, this suggests that UPF are inherently unhealthy. But that conclusion is an oversimplification of a more complex story. UPF are best viewed as being a crude indicator of unhealthy foods. The

Table 4.1 Classification of food as healthy or unhealthy using conventional food classification and NOVA system

Classification system	Categories of food	Basis of classification	Association with risk of chronic disease	Overall value of system as a tool for assessing foods and diets and for providing guidance for population
Conventional system	Healthy foods	Content of nutrients and other substances. Association of food with risk of chronic disease (mainly based on evidence from cohort studies)	Strong negative association	Strong
	Unhealthy foods	As above	Strong positive association	
NOVA System	Unprocessed/ minimally processed foods	Degree of processing	Generally associated with relatively low risk of disease (but many exceptions)	Moderate in general but may be strong for obesity
	Processed foods		Intermediate	
	Ultra-processed foods		Generally associated with relatively high risk of disease (but many exceptions)	

association between UPF and CDL is likely due to a limited number of unhealthy foods such as processed meat and sugar-sweetened beverages.

An examination of the relationship between UPF and obesity leads to an altogether different conclusion. Many UPF (but not all) are hyperpalatable and have a high energy density. As a result when people eat UPF, they are likely to consume an excessive amount of energy. When UPF constitute a major part of the diet, there is a high risk of obesity. Because obesity has such a high prevalence and is closely linked to multiple other health problems, the population should be strongly encouraged to cut their intake of UPF. This is best achieved by keeping dietary advice simple and encouraging people to eat a generally healthy diet. In addition, there is a need for policy action by governments, a concept discussed in Chap. 9.

References

1. Willett WC, Hu FB, Rimm EB, Stampfer MJ. Building better guidelines for healthy and sustainable diets. Am J Clin Nutr. 2021;114:401–42.
2. World Health Organization. Healthy Diet. 2020. https://wwwwhoint/news-room/fact-sheets/detail/healthy-diet. Accessed 14 Nov 2024.
3. Herforth A, Arimond M, Álvarez-Sánchez C, Coates J, Christianson K, Muehlhoff E. A global review of food-based dietary guidelines. Adv Nutr. 2019;10:590–605.
4. US Department of Agriculture (USDA). MyPlate. 2011. http://wwwchoosemyplategov/indexhtml. Accessed 7 Sep 2024.
5. Monteiro CA, Levy RB, Claro RM, Castro IR, Cannon G. A new classification of foods based on the extent and purpose of their processing. Cad Saúde Pública. 2010;26:2039–49.
6. Monteiro CA, Cannon G, Moubarac J-C, Levy RB, Louzada MLC, Jaime PC. The UN decade of nutrition the NOVA food classification and the trouble with ultra-processing. Public Health Nutr. 2018;21:5–17.
7. Monteiro CA, Moubarac JC, Cannon G, Ng SW, Popkin B. Ultra-processed foods: what they are and how to identify them. Public Health Nutr. 2019;22:936–41.
8. Lawrence M. Ultra-processed foods: a fit-for-purpose concept for nutrition policy activities to tackle unhealthy and unsustainable diets. Public Health Nutr. 2023;26:1384–8.
9. Ministry of Health Brazil Dietary Guidelines for the Brazilian Population, 2nd ed. 2014. Brasilia: Ministry of Health Brazil.
10. U.S. Department of Agriculture and US Department of Health and Human Services Dietary. Guidelines for Americans 2020–2025, 9th ed. 2020. https://wwwDietaryGuidelinesgov. Accessed 31 Aug 2024.
11. Temple NJ. Front-of-package food labels: a narrative review. Appetite. 2020;144:104485.
12. Julia C, Hercberg S. Development of a new front-of-pack nutrition label in France: the five-colour nutri-score. Public Health Panorama. 2017;3:712–25.
13. Sarda B, Kesse-Guyot E, Deschamps V, Ducrot P, Galan P, Hercberg S, et al. Consistency of the initial and updated version of the nutri-score with food-based dietary guidelines: a French perspective. J Nutr. 2024;154:1027–38.
14. Jacobs DR, Tapsell LC, Temple NJ. Food synergy: the key to balancing the nutrition research effort. Public Health Rev. 2011;33:509–31.
15. Caprara G. Mediterranean-type dietary pattern and physical activity: the winning combination to counteract the rising burden of non-communicable diseases (NCDs). Nutrients. 2021;13:429.
16. Forde CG. Beyond ultra-processed: considering the future role of food processing in human health. Proc Nutr Soc. 2023;82:406–18.
17. Visioli F, Marangoni F, Fogliano V, Del Rio D, Martinez JA, Kuhnle G, et al. The ultra-processed foods hypothesis: a product processed well beyond the basic ingredients in the package. Nutr Res Rev. 2023;36:340–50.
18. Temple NJ. Making sense of the relationship between ultra-processed foods obesity and other chronic diseases. Nutrients. 2024;16:4039.
19. Wolk A. Potential health hazards of eating red meat. J Intern Med. 2017;281:106–22.
20. Farvid MS, Sidahmed E, Spence ND, Mante Angua K, Rosner BA, Barnett JB. Consumption of red meat and processed meat and cancer incidence: a systematic review and meta-analysis of prospective studies. Eur J Epidemiol. 2021;36:937–51.
21. Hess JM, Comeau ME, Casperson S, Slavin JL, Johnson GH, Messina M, et al. Dietary guidelines meet NOVA: developing a menu for a healthy dietary pattern using ultra-processed foods. J Nutr. 2023;153:2472–81.
22. Lane MM, Gamage E, Du S, Ashtree DN, McGuinness AJ, Gauci S, et al. Ultra-processed food exposure and adverse health outcomes: umbrella review of epidemiological meta-analyses. BMJ. 2024;384:e077310.

23. Vitale M, Costabile G, Testa R, D'Abbronzo G, Nettore IC, Macchia PE, et al. Ultra-processed foods and human health: a systematic review and meta-analysis of prospective cohort studies. Adv Nutr. 2024;15:100121.
24. Juul F, Bere E. Ultra-processed foods – a scoping review for Nordic nutrition recommendations 2023. Food Nutr Res. 2024;24:68.
25. Temple NJ. The origins of the obesity epidemic in the USA-lessons for today. Nutrients. 2022;14:253.
26. Popkin BM, Doak CM. The obesity epidemic is a worldwide phenomenon. Nutr Rev. 1998;56(4 Pt 1):106–14.
27. Gearhardt AN, Schulte EM. Is food addictive? A review of the science. Annu Rev Nutr. 2021;41:387–410.
28. Dicken SJ, Batterham RL, Brown A. Nutrients or processing? An analysis of food and drink items from the UK National Diet and nutrition survey based on nutrient content the NOVA classification and front of package traffic light labelling. Br J Nutr. 2024;131:1619–32.
29. Klos B, Cook J, Crepaz L, Weiland A, Zipfel S, Mack I. Impact of energy density on energy intake in children and adults: a systematic review and meta-analysis of randomized controlled trials. Eur J Nutr. 2023;62:1059–76.
30. Hall KD, Ayuketah A, Brychta R, Cai H, Cassimatis T, Chen KY, et al. Ultra-processed diets cause excess calorie intake and weight gain: an inpatient randomized controlled trial of ad libitum food intake. Cell Metab. 2019;30:67–77.e3.

Healthier Alternatives to the Western Diet

5

Jasmine Chen and Karen Davison

Abstract

- The modern Western diet has contributed to the marked rise in chronic diseases of lifestyle (CDL) related to physical, mental, and cognitive health.
- Various health-promoting diet alternatives, such as the Mediterranean, DASH, Nordic, Portfolio, and vegetarian diets, have been investigated in relation to different health outcomes.
- Dietary approaches that mitigate both CDL risk and environmental impact, such as the planetary health diet, have also been considered.
- A comprehensive understanding of healthier alternatives to the Western diet combined with strategies to appropriately integrate them into the lives of different populations may help optimize human and environmental health.

Introduction: The Western Diet and Global Health

Chronic diseases of lifestyle (CDL) are among the leading causes of death and disability worldwide [1]. Major types include cardiovascular and respiratory diseases, cancer, type 2 diabetes (T2D), obesity, musculoskeletal disorders, depressive and anxiety disorders, cognitive decline, and dementias. It has been established that

J. Chen
Department of Public Health and Social Policy, University of Victoria, Victoria, BC, Canada
e-mail: jaschen@uvic.ca

K. Davison (✉)
Institute for Life Course and Aging, University of Toronto & The Centre of Clinical Excellence, Toronto, ON, Canada

Centre for Science, Athabasca University, Athabasca, AB, Canada
e-mail: karend@athabascau.ca

N. J. Temple, T. Wilson (eds.), *Pocket Primer for Nutritional Health*,
https://doi.org/10.1007/978-3-032-25402-3_5

increasingly Westernized dietary patterns are major contributors to the global burden of CDL [2], though genetic and environmental factors also play a role.

The Western diet is a modern dietary pattern characterized by high intakes of energy-dense, nutrient-poor foods, such as fast foods, soft drinks, and highly processed foods that contain relatively high amounts of added sugars, salt, and saturated fat. Figure 5.1 illustrates the typical content of a Western diet consumed in Australia with estimated cost shown in US dollars. Examples of "Western diet countries", where 65–70% of calories consumed are from animal foods, oils, fats, and sweeteners, include the United States (US), Australia, and several European countries [3]. Consequences of the Western diet range from influences on epigenetic mechanisms, nutrient availability, cofactor supply, hormone levels, cellular signaling pathways [3], oxidative stress, immune dysregulation, persistent low-grade inflammation, intestinal microbiota dysbiosis, and altered microbiota-gut-brain axis communication, to intergenerational and transgenerational effects [4].

Organizations that shape nutrition policies at national and international levels, such as the World Health Organization and the United States Department of Health and Human Services, recommend diets which balance energy intake, limit saturated and trans fats, sugar, and salt and emphasize consumption of fruits, vegetables, whole grains, and unsaturated fats. These nutrition targets may be achieved when people follow health-promoting diets, such as the Mediterranean, Dietary Approaches to Stop Hypertension (DASH), portfolio, or Nordic diets (Table 5.1). Other nutrition interventions, such as a vegetarian diet or the planetary health diet, may also lower the environmental impact. An understanding of the attributes and

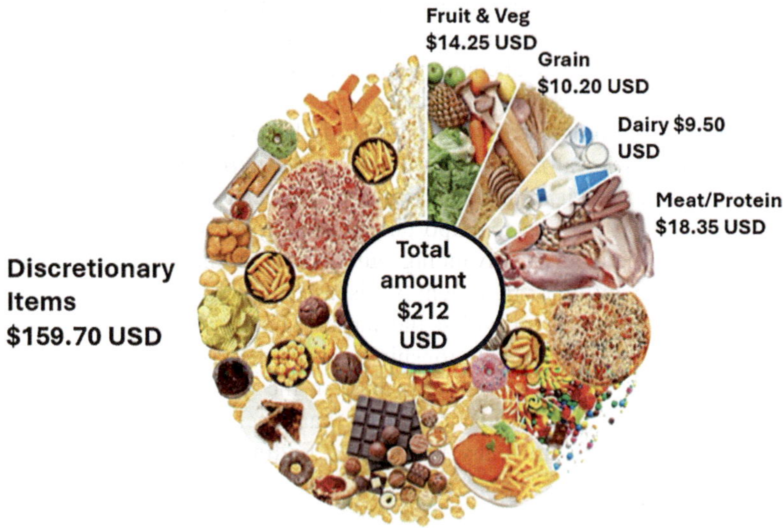

Fig. 5.1 Weekly estimated food basket distribution of Western diet [5]. (Adapted from: University of South Australia (2023). The Mediterranean Diet: Good for your health and your hip pocket. *USD* United States dollars (2023 conversion from Australian currency))

Table 5.1 Characteristics of diets that promote health and/or environmental sustainability

Mediterranean [7]	DASH[a] [8]	Portfolio [9]	MIND [10]	Healthy Nordic [11]	Vegetarian [12]	Planetary health [13]
Plant-based foods						
F: 1–2 + V: ≥2 svgs/meal Potatoes: ≤3 svgs/wk WGs: 1–2 svgs/meal Olives/nuts/seeds: 1–2 svgs/d Legumes: ≥2 svgs/wk	F/V: 4–5 svgs/d (each) WGs: 7–8 svgs/d Nuts, seeds, legumes: 4–5 svgs/wk	F/V daily Soluble viscous fiber: ≥10 g/d Nuts & soy protein: ≥30 g/d (each)	F/V daily. Berries: ≥2 & green leafy V: ≥6 svgs/wk WG: ≥3 svgs/d Nuts: ≥5 svgs/wk Beans: >3 svgs/wk	F/V: ≥500 g/d Juice: 0.4 L/wk WG Bread: 4–6 & Cereals: 1.5 svgs/d Pasta: 3 svgs/wk. ß-glucan-rich: 3 g/d Nuts (mainly almonds): 15 g/d	Flexitarian & Lacto-Ovo: Emphasize plants Pescatarian: Emphasize plants; 1/3 F/V Vegan: Plant-based; 2/3 legumes + 1/3 F/V All types emphasize WGs	F/V: 50% of total diet; 5% from starchy vegetables WGs: 15% of total diet Nuts, seeds, legumes: 15% of total diet
Animal-based foods						
LF dairy: 2 svgs/d RM <3 & White 2 svgs/wk; F/SF: ≥2 svgs/wk Eggs: 2–4 eggs/wk	LF or NF dairy: 2–3 svgs/d Lean protein: ≤2 svgs/d	Avoid: full-fat dairy, red/processed meats	Cheese: <1 svg/wk Butter: <1 Tbsp/d RM: <4 svgs/wk Poultry: ≥2 svgs/wk F/SF: ≥1 svg/wk	LF milk: ≤0.5 L/d. Cheese in cooking RM ≤500 & Poultry ≤300 g/wk F/SF: 3–5 svgs/wk Eggs: Recommended cholesterol intake	Flexitarian: Moderate & diverse sources Lacto-Ovo: Dairy & eggs only Pescatarian: 2/3 fish & seafood Vegan: No animal sources	Dairy: 4% of total diet Animal proteins: 5% of total diet

(continued)

Table 5.1 (continued)

Mediterranean [7]	DASH[a] [8]	Portfolio [9]	MIND [10]	Healthy Nordic [11]	Vegetarian [12]	Planetary health [13]
Other guidance (e.g., fats, oils, sweets, alcohol)						
Olive oil: 1–2 svgs/meal Sweets: ≤2 svgs/wk Wine: moderation	F/Os: 2–3 svgs/d Sweets: ≤5 svgs/wk Alcohol: Men ≤2, women ≤1 drink/d Sodium: <2300 mg/d	Avoid: Trans & saturated fats, processed foods & sugary beverages Plant sterols: 1–2 g/d	Olive oil mainly Sweets <5 svg/wk Fried/fast food: <1 svg/wk Alcohol: 1 drink/d	F/Os: 5 g/bread slice; 50 mL/d dressing Sweets: weekends Alcohol: Habitual amount	–	Added sugars: <5% of total diet Saturated oils/trans fats: <3.5% of total diet

Foods: *F* fruit, *F/O* fats and oils, *F/SF* fish and seafood, *LF* low fat, *NF* non-fat, *RM* red meat, *V* vegetables, *WG* whole grains. Amounts/frequency: *d* day, *g* grams, *svgs* servings, *wk* week

[a]Based on 2000 calories/d

evidence related to these diets can help advance appropriately targeted initiatives to enhance human health.

Health-Promoting Diet Alternatives: Features and Evidence

Overview of Health-Promoting Diet Alternatives

Health-promoting diet alternatives feature plant-based foods with a major emphasis on fruit, vegetables, whole grains, soya, legumes, nuts, and seeds. They may also include animal sources such as fish and seafood. These diet alternatives are good sources of phytochemicals and essential fats. Moreover, the foods which are emphasized are only minor components of ultra-processed foods [6]. Health-promoting diets may be based on certain regions, a synthesis of evidence from research, considerations of the environmental impact of the diets, or any combination of these. Table 5.1 outlines the components of different health-promoting diet alternatives. These diets are then discussed in more detail.

The Mediterranean Diet

The Mediterranean diet (MD) is based on the traditional dietary patterns of Euro-Mediterranean countries. It considers food types consumed, contributions to daily nutrient intake, food sources (e.g., sustainability) and preparation, lifestyle (e.g., physical activity), and participating in fellowship when preparing and sharing meals [7]. Variations of the MD, based on factors such as geography, culture, and religion, are reflected in the emphasis of traditional and local food products. For example, pasta consumption is higher in Italy while fish intake is higher in Spain. The number of suggested servings for food groups such as vegetables, fruits, cereals, and olive oil also varies among regions. Despite these differences, the nutrient profiles are similar.

The health-promoting MD pyramid emphasizes fiber-rich sources and various fruits and vegetables of different colors and textures. Olive oil is the primary dietary fat and is complemented with olives, nuts, seeds, and legumes. Water (1.5–2.0 L/day) is recommended, whereas wine and other fermented alcoholic beverages are permitted in moderation and to be mostly consumed with meals. Fish, white meat, eggs, and legumes are the primary protein sources. More recent versions of the MD pyramid promote environmental health by emphasizing foods derived from eco-friendly production methods that preserve the landscape and the sea [7].

The cardiovascular-related benefits of the MD were first described in the 1960s [7]. Since that time extensive investigations have been undertaken and syntheses of the evidence from systematic reviews and meta-analyses have examined the MD in relation to primary and secondary prevention of cardiovascular disease (CVD). This research leads to the conclusion that the diet can reduce the risk of fatal CVD by at least 10% and non-fatal risk by at least 21% [14].

In addition to the widely recognized cardiovascular benefits of the MD, the diet has been reported to reduce risk of other chronic diseases, improve physical and mental well-being, quality of life, and environmental sustainability. Umbrella reviews of systematic reviews with meta-analyses have reported inverse associations between the MD and all-cause mortality, cancer [15], total breast cancer (with more consistent results found among post-menopausal women [16]), mortality among colorectal and prostate cancer survivors [17], T2D [18], and neurodegenerative diseases [15]. Various systematic reviews have reported that the MD significantly reduces depressive symptoms among young and middle-aged adults with major depression or mild-to-moderate depressive symptoms [19], lowers incident frailty risk [20], decreases pain severity among those experiencing chronic musculoskeletal pain [21], slows cognitive decline [22], significantly improves health-related quality of life [23], and is positively associated with female fertility and gestational weight management [24]. Adherence to the MD may be associated with epigenetic modification of genes related to inflammation, immunocompetence, and signal transduction [25]; however, further investigation is needed to clarify the epigenetic mechanisms through which bioactive compounds of the MD exert their activity. Other research related to the sustainability of the MD suggest that it lowers greenhouse gas emissions (GHGE), water footprint, and land use [26].

Dietary Approaches to Stop Hypertension (DASH)

The DASH dietary architecture emphasizes nutrient-dense whole foods including colorful produce, legumes, unrefined grains, reduced-fat dairy products, and moderate amounts of lean protein portions from poultry, fish, and nuts [27]. This framework minimizes processed sugars, saturated fatty acids, sodium, and alcohol while optimizing dietary fiber and essential minerals such as potassium, magnesium, and calcium. For further reductions in blood pressure (BP), sodium intake of 1200 mg or less per day is suggested.

The DASH diet was the result of research in the 1990s that searched for dietary interventions to lower BP [28]. The findings showed that individuals who consumed a diet rich in fruits, vegetables, and low-fat dairy and lower in saturated and total fat and cholesterol experienced significantly larger reductions in BP than those who consumed a typical American diet. Moreover, the new diet was more effective than a diet rich in fruits and vegetables with reduced amounts of snacks and sweets. A subsequent study (DASH-Sodium) demonstrated that the DASH diet achieved a larger reduction in BP when its salt content was reduced. Later research studies reported various benefits of the DASH diet that include BP reduction among adults with and without hypertension (HT) [29], lower levels of low-density lipoprotein cholesterol (LDL-C) and total cholesterol, reduced risk of overweight/obesity, metabolic syndrome (MetS), CVD, T2D risk [30, 31], and depression [32], as well as improved pregnancy outcomes in women with gestational diabetes [33]. Children and adolescents with higher DASH scores may have lower cardiometabolic risk, but results have wide fluctuation worldwide [34]. Adherence to the DASH diet has also been reported to be negatively correlated with dietary GHGE in the USA [35].

Portfolio Diet

The portfolio diet (PD) was developed by researchers at the University of Toronto in the early 2000s. It is a vegetarian style of eating that highlights tree nuts or peanuts, plant protein (soy products or dietary pulses), viscous soluble fiber (oats, barley, eggplant, apples, oranges, berries), and plant sterols (e.g., margarine enriched with plant sterols). The main goal of the diet is to lower LDL-C. Consuming this "portfolio" of foods, partially or in their entirety, can confer cardiovascular benefit [36]. In cohort studies, systematic reviews, and meta-analyses [37–39], the PD was found to be associated with lower risk of CVD, CHD, incident T2D, and all-cause mortality as well as lower levels of LCL-C, total cholesterol, triglycerides, apolipoprotein B, C-reactive protein (CRP), and BP.

Nordic Diet

The Nordic diet (ND) and its variations (e.g., Healthy Nordic Diet, Baltic Sea Diet, New Nordic Diet) are based on common health-promoting diets (e.g., MD, DASH) and eating traditions of the Nordic countries with emphasis on food sources from plants, seas, lakes, and the wild countryside [11]. A general ND pattern includes generous amounts of green leafy and other vegetables, fruit, fish and seafood, potatoes, berries, whole grains, nuts, low-fat dairy products, vegetable oils (canola, sunflower, soya), but limited amounts of red meat and sugar.

Various ND-based studies have shown positive health outcomes. A study conducted in children reported improvements in n-3 fatty acid status with the ND that were associated with improved school performance [40]. A systematic review and dose-response analysis of cohort studies reported that higher ND adherence was associated with lower risk of all-cause, cardiovascular, and cancer mortality, as well as T2D [41]. In another systematic review with meta-analyses of cohort studies and RCTs, it was reported that ND patterns were associated with reductions in CVD incidence and mortality and T2D. Synthesis of RCT evidence indicated reductions in LDL-C, apolipoprotein B, insulin, BMI, and systolic BP [42]. Another systematic review that focused on Alzheimer's disease and dementias suggested that high ND adherence was associated with improved cognitive function [43]. The ND may also reduce risk of frailty but more investigative work is needed [44].

Mediterranean-Dash Intervention for Neurodegenerative Delay (MIND)

The MIND diet is a heart-healthy eating plan that integrates the MD and DASH diets with the goal of reducing the risk of cognitive impairments and dementia [10]. It focuses on fruit, vegetables (especially green leafy types), nuts, berries, beans, whole grains, fish, poultry, olive oil, and wine in moderation. Red meat and other foods high in total and saturated fats (butter, margarine, cheese, pastries, sweets, fried or fast food) are limited.

Several investigations suggest that the MIND diet has both cognitive and physical benefits. Systematic reviews of observational evidence have reported that higher MIND diet adherence is protective against dementia in most cohorts. However, results related to memory decline, Parkinson's disease, and brain pathology [45] were inconclusive. When RCTs of the Mediterranean, ketogenic, and MIND diets for aging populations are compared, the MIND diet shows beneficial effects related to working memory, verbal recognition, and attention in obese individuals [46]. When compared to other plant-rich diets (i.e., Mediterranean, DASH, Pro-Vegetarian, Baltic Sea), adherence to the MIND diet was superior for improving cognition [47]. A systematic review that focused on dementia risk and clinical cognitive function suggests benefits of the MIND diet for global cognition, memory, and executive function [48]. A systematic review of observational studies and RCTs that focused on cardiometabolic outcomes [49] and a scoping review that examined health outcomes other than cognition and cardiometabolic disease [50] reported that the MIND diet was associated with improvement in anthropometrics, BP, blood glucose, blood lipids, and inflammation, reduced risk of stroke, all-cause mortality, diabetes and metabolic disorders, frailty, functional ability, breast cancer, and Parkinson's disease.

Diets Consumed in Asian Cultures

In addition to the diets previously discussed, there may be others that provide health benefits among different cultural groups. Most research of dietary indexes and health outcomes focus on measures such as the MD or DASH diet score. When these have been examined among different cultures, there has been wide variation in results suggesting a bias of results among those of other ethnicities [51]. Of particular note, diets among cultures across East, Southeast, and South Asia may also contribute to the prevention and management of CDL. These diets share common features including emphasis on plant-based foods (i.e., vegetables, fruit), protein from fish, seafood, soy, legumes, nuts, whole grains (e.g., millet, barley), fermented foods, various herbs and spices, and healthy oils [52].

A meta-analysis which compared high-quality dietary patterns subdivided by animal-based, non-Asian, Asian, and plant-based indexes reported that those with increased adherence to high-quality Asian indexes had lower CVD risk [53]. The Traditional Balanced Korean diet, comprised of rice and other whole grains, fermented food, indigenous land and sea vegetables, proteins primarily from legumes and fish, herbs, and sesame and perilla oils may reduce risk of MetS, obesity, HT, and hypertriglyceridemia [54]. The traditional Chinese diet features rice or noodles, soups, vegetables, steamed breads or dumplings, fruit, vegetables, soy, seafood, and meat. In a cohort of the China Health and Nutrition Survey, where diet quality indices such as the Chinese Healthy Eating Index (CHEI) and energy-adjusted Dietary Inflammatory Index (E-DII) were considered, the risk of all-cause mortality was lowest among those with higher CHEI scores [55]. By contrast, no significant association was found between E-DII and mortality.

The traditional Japanese diet includes small portions of multiple components including rice, fish (often raw), soups, pickles, fermented soybean paste as soup base, and other ingredients such as seaweed, fruit, vegetables, and mushrooms [56]. Investigations of this diet suggest a significant inverse association with all-cause mortality and an improved healthy life expectancy [57]. Because Asian diets are biogeographically diverse, more research is needed to elucidate their health impacts.

Diets That Promote Health and Environmental Sustainability

Vegetarian Diets

Plant-based dietary patterns, such as the MD, are distinct from vegetarian diets as they do not exclude foods of animal origin [60]. Common vegetarian diet options include flexitarian, pescatarian, lacto-ovo, and vegan diets that provide varying abundance of diverse bioactive components. Individuals may select these diets for religious reasons, concerns about health, ethics, animal welfare, financial cost, environmental impact, or simply as a preference. The flexitarian diet is characterized by eating plant-based foods, varying amounts of fish and dairy, and lower quantities of meat. The diet can be adapted to dietary needs, preferences, and cultures. The pescatarian diet includes fish and shellfish but excludes meat including poultry. Those who follow a lacto-ovo vegetarian diet include dairy products and eggs but exclude meat, poultry, and fish. The vegan diet, which is the strictest, excludes all animal-derived products. These diets must be well-planned to ensure nutritional adequacy.

There has been longstanding research support for vegetarian diets, including systematic reviews. Vegetarian dietary patterns have been associated with positive effects for metabolic health, BMI, CVD, mortality risk, cancer, gut microbiome composition, and inflammation [58–61]. In another systematic review/meta-analysis, avoidance of meat was inversely associated with reduced risk of depression. However, the findings related to flexitarian diets were inconclusive [62]. A critical review that explored vegetarian diets and neurological health suggested that well-planned diets may help to reduce CRP, interleukin-6, systemic inflammation, and oxidative stress [63]. However, some vegetarian diets may be inadequate in vitamin B12, DHA, EPA, and iron which are critical to cognition and mood [64]. Although the global adoption of vegetarian diets has been growing, in countries such as the United Kingdom, the USA, Germany, and Australia, less than 12% of their populations follow these diets [65].

The evidence concerning the health and environmental impact of vegetarian diets varies between countries with the most noted effects seen in high- and middle-income countries. However, in low-income countries when food systems diversify, resource use may increase [66]. Some studies have compared the health effects of different diets with their environmental effects. Studies that compared omnivore, pescatarian, and vegetarian diets based on Healthy Eating Index (HEI) scores and environmental impact indicators have reported higher HEI scores among pescatarian and vegetarian diets, lower carbon footprint and water usage with the vegan diet, and higher carbon footprint scores with pescatarian diets [67]. An investigation was carried out that examined carbon footprint databases and representative meal plans in relation to the environmental and health-related impacts of the Standard American, MD, vegan, Paleo, and Keto diets. They also examined the Climatarian diet which focuses on local, seasonal, and fresh food, and avoidance of ruminant meats in order to minimize environmental impact. The findings revealed that diets with lower carbon footprints, particularly the vegan, Climatarian, and MD, also have positive effects on health [68]. In another study diet quality indexes (DQIs) from the National Health and Nutrition Examination Survey (NHANES; 2011–2018) were merged with GHGE, cumulative energy demand (CED), water scarcity footprint (WSF), land use, use of fertilizer nutrients and pesticides, and food price data. The researchers concluded that higher scores on most or all DQIs (HEI, Alternate HEI-2010, MD Score, Alternate MD Score, Healthful Plant-Based Diet Index (hPDI), PHD Index for the United States (PHDI), DASH Index, and Nutrient-Rich Foods Index 9.3) were associated with lower per capita CHGE, CED, land use, and use of fertilizer nutrients [69]. Conversely, all DQIs were associated with greater WSF and diet cost. The aHEI-2010 and hPDI were associated with the highest ratio of favorable-to-unfavorable sustainability outcomes. While all diets that achieve a higher DQIs have environmental trade-offs, those that place more emphasis on plant-based foods tend to have more favorable sustainability outcomes.

Clearly, further rigorous investigations that ascertain mechanistic pathways, include diverse populations, and provide health and environment-related metrics are needed to better understand the impact of vegetarian diets on the prevention and management of CDL and environmental health. However, there is now a strong case that nutrition education messaging should include recommendations toward consuming more plant-based foods, mitigating food waste, limiting consumption of ultra-processed foods, supporting local food systems, and selecting sustainable seafood [70].

Planetary Health Diet

The planetary health diet (PHD) was developed by the EAT-Lancet Commission on Food, Planet, Health [71]. The diet is based on a paper published in *The Lancet* in 2019 which attracted enormous attention and helped lead to a paradigm shift in thinking on the subject. The PHD includes a range of intakes by food groups and restricts highly processed and animal-source foods. The goals are to reduce both CDL risk and environmental degradation. The PHD considers future challenges where by 2064 global food systems will need to produce nourishing diets for nearly 9.7 billion people. Food systems are not only a major cause of CDL but also cause substantial anthropogenic GHGE [72] and freshwater withdrawals. Recent investigations also suggest that the co-occurrence of negative environmental impacts, such as long-term exposure to air pollution and underlying systemic inflammation exacerbate metabolic dysmetabolism [73]. The conversion of natural ecosystems to agricultural land also accelerates species extinction [74]. In 2025, the EAT = Lancet commission published an extensive update of the various nutritional and environmental factors related to current diets and the PHD [75].

Several investigations of the PHD have been undertaken. In an analysis of the Nurses' Health Studies (I and II) and men from the Health Professionals Follow-up Study (1986–2016), it was reported that PHD adherence was associated with lower CVD risk [76]. Similar findings were found in analyses of UK Biobank data [77]. A systematic review that assessed incident CDL risks and environmental sustainability indicators [78] reported that high PHD adherence was associated with lower T2D incidence, CVD risk markers, obesity, and environmental impact. Another systematic review of 28 case-control and cohort studies reported that higher adherence to the PHD was inversely associated with diabetes as well as CVD, cancer, and all-cause mortality [79]. Analysis of cohort data from the Black Women's Healthy Study (2001 to 2019) concluded that women with the highest adherence to the PHD had significantly lower risk of CVD mortality and all-cause mortality [80].

A criticism of the PHD is that it was developed by scientists and did not include all stakeholders affected by such dietary changes. In addition, it may not provide adequate amounts of vitamins A, B9, and B12, calcium, iron, and zinc [81]. Given the complexity of global food systems, greater unification across society, governments, academia, and civil society will be needed to define and implement planetary health initiatives.

Conclusions

The healthier alternatives to the Western diet share common themes related to their emphasis on plant foods, particularly fruit, vegetables, and whole grains. These diets typically have a high content of fiber, micronutrients, and phytochemicals. An impressive weight of evidence consistently shows that these diets are effective for the prevention and management of CDL related to physical, mental, and cognitive health. Some diets, such as the ND, PHD, and Asian Heritage Diets, need further investigation.

Educators, practitioners, and policymakers may draw upon these diets and their supporting evidence to promote health among specific populations. However, challenges are likely to persist in persuading different populations to adopt these diets. Further work is needed to ascertain their applicability in the context of factors such as food intake timing and chrononutrition [82, 83], genetics, human gut microbiome, cultural differences, socio-economics, and individual preferences. In addition, research is needed to determine if the recommended diets can be widely adopted by the global population while simultaneously achieving a strongly positive impact on the environment.

References

1. GBD 2021 Diseases and Injuries Collaborators. Global incidence, prevalence, years lived with disability (YLDs), disability-adjusted life-years (DALYs), and healthy life expectancy (HALE) for 371 diseases and injuries in 204 countries and territories and 811 subnational locations, 1990–2021: A systematic analysis for the Global Burden of Disease Study 2021. Lancet. 2024;403(10440):2133–61. https://doi.org/10.1016/S0140-6736(24)00757-8.

2. Ma H, Wang M, Qin C, Shi Y, Mandizadza OO, Ni H, Ji C. Trends in the burden of chronic diseases attributable to diet-related risk factors from 1990 to 2021 and the global projections through 2030: a population-based study. Front Nutr. 2025;12:1570321.
3. Clemente-Suárez VJ, Beltrán-Velasco AI, Redondo-Flórez L, Martín-Rodríguez A, Tornero-Aguilera JF. Global impacts of Western diet and its effects on metabolism and health: a narrative review. Nutrients. 2023;15:2749.
4. Cinquina V, Calvigioni D, Farlik M, Halbritter F, Fife-Gernedl V, Shirran SL, et al. Life-long epigenetic programming of cortical architecture by maternal 'Western' diet during pregnancy. Mol Psychiatry. 2020;25:22–36.
5. University of South Australia. The Mediterranean diet: good for your health and your hip pocket [Internet]. Adelaide: University of South Australia; 2023. https://www.unisa.edu.au/media-centre/Releases/2023/the-mediterranean-diet-good-for-your-health-and-your-hip-pocket. Accessed 12 Aug 2025.
6. Dean E, Xu J, Jones AY, Vongsirinavarat M, Lomi C, Kumar P, Ngeh E, et al. An unbiased, sustainable, evidence-informed Universal Food Guide: a timely template for national food guides. Nutr J. 2024;23:126.
7. Serra-Majem L, Tomaino L, Dernini S, Berry EM, Lairon D, Ngo de la Cruz J, et al. Updating the Mediterranean diet pyramid towards sustainability: focus on environmental concerns. Int J Environ Res Public Health. 2020;17:8758.
8. Steinberg D, Bennett GG, Svetkey L. The DASH Diet, 20 years later. JAMA. 2017;317:1529–30.
9. Portfoliodiet.org. Portfolio diet your path to heart health [Internet]. Portfoliodiet.org; 2025. https://www.portfoliodiet.org. Accessed 12 Aug 2025.
10. Marcason W. What are the components to the MIND diet? J Acad Nutr Diet. 2015;115:1744.
11. Adamsson V, Reumark A, Cederholm T, Vessby B, Riserus U, Johansson G. What is a healthy Nordic diet? Foods and nutrients in the NORDIET study. Food Nutr Res. 2012;56:1–8.
12. Guest NS, Raj S, Landry MJ, Mangels AR, Pawlak R, Senkus KE, et al. Vegetarian and vegan dietary patterns to treat adult type 2 diabetes: a systematic review and meta-analysis of randomized controlled trials. Adv Nutr. 2024;15:100294.
13. EAT. The planetary health diet [Internet]. EAT; 2025. https://eatforum.org/eat-lancet-commission/the-planetary-health-diet-and-you. Accessed 12 Aug 2025.
14. Hareer LW, Lau YY, Mole F, Reidlinger DP, O'Neill HM, Mayr HL, et al. The effectiveness of the Mediterranean diet for primary and secondary prevention of cardiovascular disease: an umbrella review. Nutr Diet. 2025;82:8–41.
15. Dinu M, Pagliai G, Casini A, Sofi F. Mediterranean diet and multiple health outcomes: an umbrella review of meta-analyses of observational studies and randomised trials. Eur J Clin Nutr. 2018;72:30–43.
16. González-Palacios Torres C, Barrios-Rodríguez R, Muñoz-Bravo C, Toledo E, Dierssen T, Jiménez-Moleón JJ. Mediterranean diet and risk of breast cancer: an umbrella review. Clin Nutr. 2023;42:600–8.
17. Castro-Espin C, Agudo A. The role of diet in prognosis among cancer survivors: a systematic review and meta-analysis of dietary patterns and diet interventions. Nutrients. 2022;14:348.
18. Zhang Y, Yang Y, Huang Q, Zhang Q, Li M, Wu Y. The effectiveness of lifestyle interventions for diabetes remission on patients with type 2 diabetes mellitus: a systematic review and meta-analysis. Worldviews Evid-Based Nurs. 2023;20:64–78.
19. Bizzozero-Peroni B, Martínez-Vizcaíno V, Fernández-Rodríguez R, Jiménez-López E, Núñez de Arenas-Arroyo S, Saz-Lara A, et al. The impact of the Mediterranean diet on alleviating depressive symptoms in adults: a systematic review and meta-analysis of randomized controlled trials. Nutr Rev. 2025;83:29–39.
20. Dominguez LJ, Donat-Vargas C, Sayon-Orea C, Barberia-Latasa M, Veronese N, Rey-Garcia J, et al. Rationale of the association between Mediterranean diet and the risk of frailty in older adults and systematic review and meta-analysis. Exp Gerontol. 2023;177:112180.
21. Cuevas-Cervera M, Perez-Montilla JJ, Gonzalez-Muñoz A, Garcia-Rios MC, Navarro-Ledesma S. The effectiveness of intermittent fasting, time restricted feeding, caloric restriction, a ketogenic diet and the Mediterranean diet as part of the treatment plan to improve

health and chronic musculoskeletal pain: a systematic review. Int J Environ Res Public Health. 2022;19:6698.
22. Devranis P, Vassilopoulou E, Tsironis V, Sotiriadis PM, Chourdakis M, Aivaliotis M, et al. Mediterranean diet, ketogenic diet or MIND diet for aging populations with cognitive decline: a systematic review. Life (Basel). 2023;13:173.
23. Godos J, Guglielmetti M, Ferraris C, Frias-Toral E, Domínguez Azpíroz I, Lipari V, et al. Mediterranean diet and quality of life in adults: a systematic review. Nutrients. 2025;17:577.
24. Yang J, Song Y, Gaskins AJ, Li LJ, Huang Z, Eriksson JG, et al. Mediterranean diet and female reproductive health over lifespan: a systematic review and meta-analysis. Am J Obstet Gynecol. 2023;229:617–31.
25. Caprara G. Mediterranean-type dietary pattern and physical activity: the winning combination to counteract the rising burden of non-communicable diseases (NCDs). Nutrients. 2021;13:429.
26. Lorca-Camara V, Bosque-Prous M, Bes-Rastrollo M, O'Callaghan-Gordo C, Bach-Faig A. Environmental and health sustainability of the Mediterranean diet: a systematic review. Adv Nutr. 2024;15:100322.
27. Chiavaroli L, Viguiliouk E, Nishi SK, Blanco Mejia S, Rahelić D, Kahleová H, et al. DASH dietary pattern and cardiometabolic outcomes: an umbrella review of systematic reviews and meta-analyses. Nutrients. 2019;11:338.
28. Filippou CD, Tsioufis CP, Thomopoulos CG, Mihas CC, Dimitriadis KS, Sotiropoulou LI, et al. Dietary Approaches to Stop Hypertension (DASH) diet and blood pressure reduction in adults with and without hypertension: a systematic review and meta-analysis of randomized controlled trials. Adv Nutr. 2020;11:1150–60.
29. Theodoridis X, Chourdakis M, Chrysoula L, Chroni V, Tirodimos I, Dipla K, et al. Adherence to the DASH diet and risk of hypertension: a systematic review and meta-analysis. Nutrients. 2023;15:3261.
30. Lari A, Sohouli MH, Fatahi S, Cerqueira HS, Santos HO, Pourrajab B, et al. The effects of the Dietary Approaches to Stop Hypertension (DASH) diet on metabolic risk factors in patients with chronic disease: a systematic review and meta-analysis of randomized controlled trials. Nutr Metab Cardiovasc Dis. 2021;31:2766–78.
31. Valenzuela-Fuenzalida JJ, Bravo VS, Valarezo LM, Delgado Retamal MF, Leiva JM, Bruna-Mejías A, et al. Effectiveness of DASH diet versus other diet modalities in patients with metabolic syndrome: a systematic review and meta-analysis. Nutrients. 2024;16:3054.
32. Tan J, Wang C, Tomiyama AJ. Dietary Approaches to Stop Hypertension (DASH) diet and mental well-being: a systematic review. Nutr Rev. 2023;82:60–75.
33. Di J, Fan J, Ma F. Comparative efficacy of dietary interventions for glycemic control and pregnancy outcomes in gestational diabetes: a network meta-analysis of randomized controlled trials. Front Endocrinol (Lausanne). 2025;16:1512493.
34. Teixeira B, Afonso C, Rodrigues S, Oliveira A. Healthy and sustainable dietary patterns in children and adolescents: a systematic review. Adv Nutr. 2022;13:1144–85.
35. Frank SM, Jaacks LM, Meyer K, Rose D, Adair LS, Avery CL, et al. Dietary quality and dietary greenhouse gas emissions in the USA: a comparison of the planetary health diet index, healthy eating index-2015, and dietary approaches to stop hypertension. Int J Behav Nutr Phys Act. 2024;21:36.
36. Glenn AJ, Guasch-Ferré M, Malik VS, Kendall CWC, Manson JE, Rimm EB, et al. Portfolio diet score and risk of cardiovascular disease: findings from 3 prospective cohort studies. Circulation. 2023;148:1750–63.
37. Chatzi CA, Basios A, Markozannes G, Ntzani EE, Tsilidis KK, Kazakos K, et al. Effect of different dietary patterns on cardiometabolic risk factors: an umbrella review of systematic reviews and meta-analyses. Nutrients. 2024;16:3873.
38. Kahleova H, Salas-Salvadó J, Rahelić D, Kendall CW, Rembert E, Sievenpiper JL. Dietary patterns and cardiometabolic outcomes in diabetes: a summary of systematic reviews and meta-analyses. Nutrients. 2019;11:2209.

39. Glenn AJ, Hernández-Alonso P, Kendall CWC, Martínez-González MÁ, Corella D, Fitó M, et al. Longitudinal changes in adherence to the portfolio and DASH dietary patterns and cardiometabolic risk factors in the PREDIMED-Plus study. Clin Nutr. 2021;40:2825–36.
40. Sørensen LB, Damsgaard CT, Dalskov SM, Petersen RA, Egelund N, Dyssegaard CB, et al. Diet-induced changes in iron and n-3 fatty acid status and associations with cognitive performance in 8–11-year-old Danish children: secondary analyses of the Optimal Well-Being, Development and Health for Danish Children through a Healthy New Nordic Diet School Meal Study. Br J Nutr. 2015;114:1623–37.
41. Jalilpiran Y, Jayedi A, Djafarian K, Shab-Bidar S. The Nordic diet and the risk of non-communicable chronic disease and mortality: a systematic review and dose-response meta-analysis of prospective cohort studies. Crit Rev Food Sci Nutr. 2022;62:3124–36.
42. Massara P, Zurbau A, Glenn AJ, Chiavaroli L, Khan TA, Viguiliouk E, et al. Nordic dietary patterns and cardiometabolic outcomes: a systematic review and meta-analysis of prospective cohort studies and randomised controlled trials. Diabetologia. 2022;65:2011–31.
43. Christodoulou CC, Pitsillides M, Hadjisavvas A, Zamba-Papanicolaou E. Dietary intake, Mediterranean and Nordic diet adherence in Alzheimer's disease and dementia: a systematic review. Nutrients. 2025;17:336.
44. Hanbali S, Avgerinou C. Association between adherence to the Nordic diet and frailty in older adults: a systematic review of observational studies. Maturitas. 2024;182:107923.
45. van Soest AP, Beers S, van de Rest O, de Groot LC. The Mediterranean-Dietary Approaches to Stop Hypertension Intervention for Neurodegenerative Delay (MIND) diet for the aging brain: a systematic review. Adv Nutr. 2024;15:100184.
46. Devranis P, Vassilopoulou E, Tsironis V, Sotiriadis PM, Chourdakis M, Aivaliotis M, et al. Mediterranean diet, ketogenic diet or MIND diet for aging populations with cognitive decline: a systematic review. Life (Basel, Switzerland). 2023;13:173.
47. Kheirouri S, Alizadeh M. MIND diet and cognitive performance in older adults: a systematic review. Crit Rev Food Sci Nutr. 2022;62:8059–77.
48. Tse JHW, Law QPS, Tsang JTY, Suen LKP, Tyrovolas S, Kwan RYC. The association between the MIND diet and cognitive health in middle-aged and older adults: a systematic review. J Nutr Health Aging. 2025;29:100630.
49. Akbar Z, Fituri S, Ouagueni A, Alalwani J, Sukik A, Al-Jayyousi GF, et al. Associations of the MIND diet with cardiometabolic diseases and their risk factors: a systematic review. Diabetes Metab Syndr Obes. 2023;16:3353–71.
50. Morgan KH, Lee ML, Barroso CS, Anderson JG, Lott S, Reth D, Horn C, Dixson M. Associations of the MIND diet with human health outcomes: a scoping review. Nutrients. 2025;17:2687.
51. Zheng J, Zhu T, Li F, Wu H, Jiang S, Shivappa N, et al. Diet quality and mortality among Chinese adults: findings from the China health and nutrition survey. Nutrients. 2024;16:94.
52. Oldways. What is the Asian heritage diet? [Internet]. USA: Oldways; 2025. https://oldwayspt.org/traditional-diets/asian-heritage-diet. Accessed 12 Aug 2025.
53. Lim GH, Neelakantan N, Lee YQ, Park SH, Kor ZH, van Dam RM, et al. Dietary patterns and cardiovascular diseases in Asia: a systematic review and meta-analysis. Adv Nutr. 2024;15:100249.
54. Lee KW, Cho MS. The traditional Korean dietary pattern is associated with decreased risk of metabolic syndrome: findings from the Korean National Health and Nutrition Examination Survey, 1998–2009. J Med Food. 2014;17:43–56.
55. Gabriel AS, Ninomiya K, Uneyama H. The role of the Japanese traditional diet in healthy and sustainable dietary patterns around the world. Nutrients. 2018;10:173.
56. Abe C, Imai T, Sezaki A, Miyamoto K, Kawase F, Shirai Y, et al. Global association between traditional Japanese diet score and all-cause, cardiovascular disease, and total cancer mortality: a cross-sectional and longitudinal ecological study. J Am Nutr Assoc. 2023;42:660–7.
57. Yannakoulia M, Scarmeas N. Diets. N Engl J Med. 2024;390:2098–106.

58. Raj S, Guest NS, Landry MJ, Mangels AR, Pawlak R, Rozga M. Vegetarian dietary patterns for adults: a position paper of the Academy of Nutrition and Dietetics. J Acad Nutr Diet. 2025;125:831–46.e2
59. Almuntashiri SA, Alsubaie FF, Alotaybi M. Plant-based diets and their role in preventive medicine: a systematic review of evidence-based insights for reducing disease risk. Cureus. 2025;17:e78629.
60. Landry MJ, Senkus KE, Mangels AR, Guest NS, Pawlak R, Raj S, et al. Vegetarian dietary patterns and cardiovascular risk factors and disease prevention: an umbrella review of systematic reviews. Am J Prev Cardiol. 2024;20:100868.
61. Ilari S, Proietti S, Milani F, Vitiello L, Muscoli C, Russo P, et al. Dietary patterns, oxidative stress, and early inflammation: a systematic review and meta-analysis comparing Mediterranean, vegan, and vegetarian diets. Nutrients. 2025;17:548.
62. Luque-Martínez A, Ávila-Jiménez ÁF, Reinoso-Espín Á, Araújo-Jiménez MÁ, Martos-Salcedo CR, González-Domenech P, et al. Meat consumption and depression: an updated systematic review and meta-analysis. Nutrients. 2025;17:811.
63. Clemente-Suárez VJ, Redondo-Flórez L, Martín-Rodríguez A, Curiel-Regueros A, Rubio-Zarapuz A, Tornero-Aguilera JF. Impact of vegan and vegetarian diets on neurological health: a critical review. Nutrients. 2025;17:884.
64. Cooreman-Algoed M, Boone L, Dewulf J, Nachtergaele P, Taelman SE, Lachat C. Environmental sustainability and nutritional quality of different diets considering nutritional adequacy. Sci Total Environ. 2024;955:176967.
65. The Vegan Society Worldwide Veganism Statistics. https://www.vegansociety.com/news/media/statistics/worldwide. Accessed 12 Aug 2025.
66. Springmann M, Wiebe K, Mason-D'Croz D, Sulser TB, Rayner M, Scarborough P. Health and nutritional aspects of sustainable diet strategies and their association with environmental impacts: a global modelling analysis with country-level detail. Lancet Planet Health. 2018;2:e451–61.
67. O'Malley K, Willits-Smith A, Rose D. Popular diets as selected by adults in the United States show wide variation in carbon footprints and diet quality. Am J Clin Nutr. 2023;117:701–8.
68. Dixon KA, Michelsen MK, Carpenter CL. Modern diets and the health of our planet: an investigation into the environmental impacts of food choices. Nutrients. 2023;15:692.
69. Conrad Z, Thorne-Lyman AL, Wu S, DiStaso C, Korol M, Love DC. Are healthier diets more sustainable? A cross-sectional assessment of 8 diet quality indexes and 7 sustainability metrics. Am J Clin Nutr. 2025;121:315–23.
70. Bastian GE, Buro D, Palmer-Keenan DM. Recommendations for integrating evidence-based, sustainable diet information into nutrition education. Nutrients. 2021;13:4170.
71. Willett W, Rockström J, Loken B, Springmann M, Lang T, Vermeulen S, et al. Food in the Anthropocene: the EAT-Lancet Commission on healthy diets from sustainable food systems. Lancet. 2019;393:447–92.
72. Food and Agriculture Organization of the United Nations. The state of the world's land and water resources for food and agriculture—systems at breaking point. Synthesis report 2021. Rome; 2021. https://openknowledge.fao.org/server/api/core/bitstreams/ecb51a59-ac4d-407a-80de-c7d6c3e15fcc/content. Accessed 12 Aug 2025.
73. Muszalska A, Wiecanowska J, Michałowska J, Pastusiak-Zgolińska KM, Polok I, Łompieś K, et al. The role of the Planetary Diet in managing metabolic syndrome and cardiovascular disease: a narrative review. Nutrients. 2025;17:862.
74. Tilman D, Clark M, Williams DR, Kimmel K, Polasky S, Packer C. Future threats to biodiversity and pathways to their prevention. Nature. 2017;546:73–81.
75. Rockström J, Thilsted SH, Willett WC, Gordon LJ, Herrero M, Hicks CC, et al. The EAT-Lancet Commission on healthy, sustainable, and just food systems. Lancet. 2025;406:1625–700.
76. Sawicki CM, Ramesh G, Bui L, Nair NK, Hu FB, Rimm EB, et al. Planetary health diet and cardiovascular disease: results from three large prospective cohort studies in the USA. Lancet Planet Health. 2024;8:e666–74.

77. Sotos-Prieto M, Ortolá R, Maroto-Rodriguez J, Carballo-Casla A, Kales SN, Rodríguez-Artalejo F. Association between planetary health diet and cardiovascular disease: a prospective study from the UK biobank. Eur J Prev Cardiol. 2025;32:394–401.
78. Ojo O, Jiang Y, Ojo OO, Wang X. The association of planetary health diet with the risk of type 2 diabetes and related complications: a systematic review. Healthcare (Basel). 2023;11:1120.
79. Liu J, Shen Q, Wang X. Emerging EAT-Lancet planetary health diet is associated with major cardiovascular diseases and all-cause mortality: a global systematic review and meta-analysis. Clin Nutr. 2024;43:167–79.
80. Shan Y, Bertrand KA, Petrick JL, Sheehy S, Palmer JR. Planetary Health Diet Index in relation to mortality in a prospective cohort study of United States black females. Am J Clin Nutr. 2025;121:589–96.
81. Beal T, Ortenzi F, Fanzo J. Estimated micronutrient shortfalls of the EAT-Lancet planetary health diet. Lancet Planet Health. 2023;7:e233–7.
82. Dai Z, Wan K, Miyashita M, Ho RS, Zheng C, Poon ET, et al. The effect of time-restricted eating combined with exercise on body composition and metabolic health: a systematic review and meta-analysis. Adv Nutr. 2024;15:100262.
83. Rovira-Llopis S, Luna-Marco C, Perea-Galera L, Bañuls C, Morillas C, Victor VM. Circadian alignment of food intake and glycaemic control by time-restricted eating: a systematic review and meta-analysis. Rev Endocr Metab Disord. 2024;25:325–37.

Dietary Supplements: What Can Be Recommended?

6

Norman J. Temple

Abstract

- Many types of dietary supplements are available for purchase and are widely used. However, the evidence demonstrating that they enhance health is mostly weak.
- Multivitamins are a popular dietary supplement but there is little evidence of their benefit to health.
- A low blood level of vitamin D is associated with an increased risk of a wide variety of diseases. There is a strong case that the general population should take a vitamin D supplement.
- Fatty fish have a high content of long-chain n-3 polyunsaturated fatty acids (marine fats). These fats have cardioprotective benefits. It is recommended that people should regularly eat fatty fish. Dietary supplements of fish oil are an alternative for people who do not consume fatty fish.
- The microbiome in the colon has a significant impact on health. Probiotics contain particular bacteria in a concentrated form. Taken as a supplement they can change the numbers of different types of bacteria in the colon. This means that probiotics can help prevent several diseases and can also act as an effective therapy.

N. J. Temple (✉)
Centre for Science, Athabasca University, Athabasca, AB, Canada
e-mail: normant@athabascau.ca

N. J. Temple, T. Wilson (eds.), *Pocket Primer for Nutritional Health*,
https://doi.org/10.1007/978-3-032-25402-3_6

Introduction

Dietary supplements refer to any substance taken in addition to regular food. Supplements include vitamins, minerals, amino acids, enzymes, and various substances extracted from plants and animals. By definition, these products are not conventional foods but are intended to supplement the diet, generally with the intent of improving health and body functioning and of preventing or treating disease. Hundreds of dietary supplements of all types are on sale to the public as is easily seen on a visit to a health food store.

Around half of adults in the USA take dietary supplements [1]. The quality of the evidence supporting their efficacy covers a wide spectrum. In order for claims to have real credibility we need to see hard scientific evidence. Ideally, there should be consistent evidence from well-conducted RCTs, with clinical endpoints, showing health benefits, and published in peer-reviewed journals. But such evidence is only available for a small minority of supplements. Nevertheless, the staff in health food stores generally have little hesitation in making highly exaggerated claims for the beneficial effects of the supplements they sell [2].

This chapter provides a brief review of a small number of supplements. The ones chosen for inclusion are those that are especially popular or that may be of value to health based on evidence of at least moderate strength.

Vitamins and Minerals

Many supplements are formulations containing one or more vitamins and/or minerals.

Multivitamins

Multivitamins is a commonly used name that refers to pills that contain a broad spectrum of vitamins and minerals and that are typically taken once a day. They are the most popular type of dietary supplement. People most likely to gain benefit from their use are those at risk of malnutrition such as people who habitually consume a low-calorie diet which is often the case with elderly people and those with anorexia, drug addiction, or advanced cancer. But what about healthy people? Much evidence has come from prospective cohort studies and from RCTs. Findings consistently reveal that people who consume a multivitamin supplement do not have a significant reduction in cancer or cardiovascular disease, or have a reduced all-cause mortality [3, 4].

Supplements During Pregnancy

A low intake of folate is also common because a large section of the population eat an unhealthy diet with a low content of nutritious foods, especially fruit and vegetables. This problem is a serious concern as it may lead to the development of a type of congenital malformation during pregnancy called neural tube defects, such as spina bifida. However, this problem is now much less common than in former times as grain products in the USA are now fortified with folic acid, a policy that was started in 1996. Other evidence indicates that a multivitamin supplement is of value during pregnancy for both the mother and the developing fetus. For that reason, women who are pregnant or may become pregnant are advised to take a supplement that contains not only folic acid but also other micronutrients.

Vitamin D

It has been well known for decades that vitamin D plays a critical role in calcium balance and bone health. Very little of the vitamin comes from the diet; the main source is the action of sunshine on the skin. The most reliable indicator of a person's vitamin D status is their blood level of the vitamin. A low blood level is a good indicator of an elevated risk of osteoporosis and therefore of bone fractures.

Starting around the year 2000, much evidence has accumulated revealing that the harmful effects of a poor vitamin D status go well beyond bone health. Prospective cohort studies have generated impressive evidence indicating that a low blood level of the vitamin is associated with an increased risk of a wide variety of diseases. In some studies, vitamin D status was measured using proxy measures namely exposure to sunshine or consumption of vitamin supplements. The diseases linked to a poor vitamin D status include many types of cancer, dementia (including Alzheimer's disease), type 2 diabetes, chronic obstructive pulmonary disease, and cardiovascular disease (CVD, including hypertension and stroke) [5–7]. A poor vitamin D status is also associated with an increased all-cause mortality and depressed immune function [6].

In contrast to the strong evidence that has come from cohort studies, a different story has emerged from RCTs. Trials of supplemental vitamin D have generated inconsistent findings. In the case of cancer, there is clear evidence of a reduction in mortality [8], but with most other diseases there is only weak evidence of health benefits. The most plausible explanation for the failure of RCTs to consistently generate evidence as to the benefit of vitamin D supplements is that the experimental design used in these studies is flawed [6].

Taking the above evidence as a whole, there is a strong case that the general population should take a vitamin D supplement. A commonly recommended dose is around 1000 IU (25 μg) per day. However, much evidence suggests that an optimal dose is likely to be double that amount [6].

The need for supplementation is especially strong in the population groups who are most likely to have low blood levels of the vitamin. These include those with inadequate skin exposure to the sun such as frail older people and inhabitants of northern latitudes, including the northern states of the USA and the whole of Canada. Persons with dark skin are especially vulnerable to deficiency.

Iron

Many women are lacking in iron during their reproductive years and may benefit from a supplement. In the case of iron, this is due to a combination of poor intake and menstrual loss which results in anemia. As meat is a rich source of iron, vegetarians are at most risk.

Calcium

Calcium is another popular supplement and is often taken by middle-aged and older women in the hope that it will help protect against osteoporosis. Findings from RCTs have been mostly negative regarding the value of this supplement [9].

Marine Fats

Many types of fish have a relatively high fat content. The fat is predominately long-chain n-3 polyunsaturated fatty acids. The two main fatty acids are eicosapentaenoic acid (EPA) and docosahexaenoic acid (DHA). These fatty acids are believed to exert several cardioprotective actions including defending against inflammation and thrombosis, and lowering the blood triglyceride level while raising HDL-cholesterol.

Meta-analyses of cohort studies have reported a significant protective association between the intake of the above fats and risk of coronary heart disease (CHD) [10, 11]. This is seen for both CHD incidence and mortality. Similar findings have been reported for type 2 diabetes and total mortality. In some cases, the dietary measurement was of fatty fish [10], while in others it was of DHA/EPA [11].

In a pooled analysis of 192,000 subjects in four cohort studies, the findings revealed that consumption of fatty fish has a protective association with both sudden cardiac death and CVD [12]. However, this was only seen in subjects who were at high risk of CVD or who already had CVD at the start of the study. No protective association was seen in persons who were initially free of CVD.

RCTs have generated findings that are consistent with the above observations. A meta-analysis was carried out of 42 RCTs that included 150,000 subjects [13]. The subjects were either at high risk of CVD or had prior CVD. A clear cardioprotective benefit was seen for intake of DHA/EPA. The cardiovascular condition where the benefit was strongest - a 35% reduction.

The first and least controversial conclusion from the above findings is that the general population should be advised to eat at least one or two servings of fatty fish per week. The optimum intake may be as much as three or four servings per week. Fatty fish includes salmon, herring, mackerel, sardines, and pilchards. There is an absence of evidence that lean fish, such as cod, halibut, and hake, provides cardioprotective benefits.

Dietary supplements of fish oil represent an alternative for people who do not consume fatty fish or only eat small amounts. Such supplements are typically rich sources of DHA and EPA. The persons most likely to benefit from supplements of fish oil are those who have CVD or are at high risk of the disease.

Probiotics

Probiotics are not technically dietary supplements but are included here as they are marketed and used much like true dietary supplements.

The study of the microbiome and its relationship to health has emerged as a hot topic in recent years. The focus has been on the bacteria present in the colon. The rationale for giving supplements of probiotics, preparations containing particular bacteria in a concentrated form, is to change the numbers of different types of bacteria in the colon in a way that enhances health. Findings from RCTs provide impressive evidence that specific probiotics have a beneficial impact on colon function which helps prevent several diseases and is therapeutic for others.

Probiotics appear to be effective for the prevention of urinary tract infections in women, respiratory tract infections, and antibiotic-associated diarrhea [14]. Consistent with this apparent protection against several types of infection, probiotics have been reported to enhance the immune response [15]. They may also improve the symptoms of persons with depression [16]. Evidence also indicates that probiotics have a beneficial effect on several risk factors for cardiovascular disease [14].

Despite this impressive evidence, responsible health authorities have not made a general recommendation that healthy people should routinely consume probiotics. The major reason for this caution is that the evidence is not yet considered sufficiently robust to justify such a recommendation. In addition, and also of great importance, the formulation of probiotics is highly variable. So, even if it becomes firmly established that, for example, probiotics prevent respiratory tract infections, this does not necessarily mean that a particular brand of probiotics bought in a health food store will achieve the same benefit. This is because the wrong type of bacteria may be included in the formulation or the dose may be wrong.

Conclusions

For decades, the subject of dietary supplements has been at the center of much controversy. But even among well-trained health professionals, there is a long history of misleading advice being given. One well-known example is that of megadoses of vitamin C. But we should not throw the baby out with the bathwater. In a limited number of cases, we have solid evidence that a supplement does provide a benefit to health. This chapter has provided a handful of examples as summarized in Table 6.1. No doubt future research will reveal more examples. Based on the information provided in Chap. 7, phytochemicals are likely to be a fertile area in this regard.

Table 6.1 Possible benefits of dietary supplements: summary

Supplement	Target group	Possible benefits	Comments
Multivitamins	Persons at risk of malnutrition	Prevention of disorders related to vitamin/mineral deficiency	Examples where multivitamins are advised include anorexia, elderly people who have a low energy intake
Multivitamins including folic acid	Pregnant women	Prevention of spina bifida. Improved health during pregnancy for both the mother and the developing fetus	Use of multivitamins should be started before pregnancy or in first few weeks
Vitamin D	General population especially persons with inadequate exposure to the sun	Multiple health benefits	
Iron	Women during reproductive years if anemia or low iron status is present	Prevention of anemia	
Calcium	Middle-aged and older women	Often claimed that it improves bone health	Not recommended due to lack of evidence
Marine fats (long-chain n-3 polyunsaturated fat)	Persons who consume little or no fatty fish	Lowers risk of CHD and sudden cardiac death. May also lower risk of type 2 diabetes and all-cause mortality	Benefit is most likely in persons at elevated risk of CVD
Probiotics	No specific target group	May lower risk of some types of infection and improve immune response. Possible benefit for other health conditions	No recommendation at present for general population or specific groups. Much uncertainty over ideal formulation (species of bacteria and dose)

References

1. Kantor ED, Rehm CD, Du M, White E. Giovannucci EL Trends in dietary supplement use among US adults from 1999-2012. JAMA. 2016;316:1464–74.
2. Temple NJ. Dietary supplements and health. One part science, nine parts hype. In: Temple NJ, Wilson T, Jacobs DR, Bray GA, editors. Nutritional health: strategies for disease prevention. 4th ed. New York: Humana Press; 2023. p. 389–400.

3. Loftfield E, O'Connell CP, Abnet CC, Graubard BI, Liao LM, Beane Freeman LE, et al. Multivitamin use and mortality risk in 3 prospective US cohorts. JAMA Netw Open. 2024;7:e2418729.
4. O'Connor EA, Evans CV, Ivlev I, Rushkin MC, Thomas RG, Martin A, et al. Vitamin and mineral supplements for the primary prevention of cardiovascular disease and cancer: updated evidence report and systematic review for the US Preventive Services Task Force. JAMA. 2022;327:2334–47.
5. Chen LJ, Sha S, Stocker H, Brenner H, Schöttker B. The associations of serum vitamin D status and vitamin D supplements use with all-cause dementia, Alzheimer's disease, and vascular dementia: a UK Biobank based prospective cohort study. Am J Clin Nutr. 2024;119:1052–64.
6. Grant WB, Wimalawansa SJ, Pludowski P, Cheng RZ. Vitamin D: evidence-based health benefits and recommendations for population guidelines. Nutrients. 2025;17:277.
7. Kiely M, Brennan L, Dunlop T, Tate G, Woodside JV, Moretti D. Working group 1 of the Federation of European Nutrition Societies (FENS) presidential activity. Prevention of chronic disease using vitamins-a case study of the vitamin D and cardiovascular disease hypothesis using evidence from randomised controlled and prospective cohort studies. Eur J Nutr. 2025;64:199.
8. Guo Z, Huang M, Fan D, Hong Y, Zhao M, Ding R, et al. Association between vitamin D supplementation and cancer incidence and mortality: a trial sequential meta-analysis of randomized controlled trials. Crit Rev Food Sci Nutr. 2023;63:8428–42.
9. Reid IR, Bolland MJ. Controversies in medicine: the role of calcium and vitamin D supplements in adults. Med J Aust. 2019;211:468–73.
10. Giosuè A, Calabrese I, Lupoli R, Riccardi G, Vaccaro O, Vitale M. Relations between the consumption of fatty or lean fish and risk of cardiovascular disease and all-cause mortality: a systematic review and meta-analysis. Adv Nutr. 2022;13:1554–65.
11. Jiang H, Wang L, Wang D, Yan N, Li C, Wu M, et al. Omega-3 polyunsaturated fatty acid biomarkers and risk of type 2 diabetes, cardiovascular disease, cancer, and mortality. Clin Nutr. 2022;41:1798–807.
12. Mohan D, Mente A, Dehghan M, et al. Associations of fish consumption with risk of cardiovascular disease and mortality among individuals with or without vascular disease from 58 countries. JAMA Intern Med. 2021;181:631–49.
13. Tutor A, O'Keefe EL, Lavie CJ, Elagizi A, Milani R, O'Keefe J. Omega-3 fatty acids in primary and secondary prevention of cardiovascular diseases. Prog Cardiovasc Dis. 2024;84:19–26.
14. Merenstein DJ, Tancredi DJ, Karl JP, Krist AH, Lenoir-Wijnkoop I, Reid G, et al. Is there evidence to support probiotic use for healthy people? Adv Nutr. 2024;15:100265.
15. You S, Ma Y, Yan B, Pei W, Wu Q, Ding C, et al. The promotion mechanism of prebiotics for probiotics: a review. Front Nutr. 2022;9:1000517.
16. Lin J, Zhang Y, Wang K, Wang J, Kou S, Chen K, et al. The effect and safety of probiotics on depression: a systematic review and meta-analysis of randomized controlled trials. Eur J Nutr. 2023;62:2709–21.

Phytochemicals in Food and Their Health Benefits

7

Rafik Assabgui and Karen Davison

Abstract

- Phytochemicals are diverse groups of natural bioactive compounds produced in plants.
- Food sources include fruits, vegetables, whole grains, nuts, legumes, seeds, and teas.
- Phytochemicals affect many areas of body functioning including gut microbiota, metabolic pathways, inflammation, antioxidant systems, and cognitive function.
- Research studies highlight their role in the prevention and management of many chronic diseases of lifestyle and communicable diseases. Some have adverse effects, such as toxicity and nutrient interference, especially if consumed in excessive amounts.
- Future investigative work is needed to discern their individual, additive, and synergistic effects in relation to human health.
- Advancements in nutrigenomics and metabolomics will further understanding of phytochemicals' applications related to health promotion.

R. Assabgui
Agriculture and Agri-Food Canada, Ottawa, ON, Canada
e-mail: Rafik.assabgui@canada.ca

K. Davison (✉)
Institute for Life Course and Aging, University of Toronto & The Centre of Clinical Excellence, Toronto, ON, Canada

Centre for Science, Athabasca University, Athabasca, AB, Canada
e-mail: karend@athabascau.ca

N. J. Temple, T. Wilson (eds.), *Pocket Primer for Nutritional Health*,
https://doi.org/10.1007/978-3-032-25402-3_7

Introduction

Plants produce and store thousands of secondary metabolites located in all parts including the stems, leaves, roots, and bark. Many of these metabolites are referred to as phytochemicals and are variably distributed in fruits, vegetables, whole grains, legumes, nuts, seeds, oils, tea, herbs, and spices. Like nutrients, phytochemicals are biologically active compounds that are metabolized, oxidized, or modified. They are not deemed essential for human health; however, diets rich in fruits, vegetables, whole grains, legumes, and other plants are associated with reduced risk of chronic diseases of lifestyle (CDL) and communicable diseases. In addition, their potential for therapeutic applications is an area of ongoing research.

Much of the evidence referred to in this chapter is based on epidemiological studies, especially prospective cohort studies. These have consistently shown that intake of whole foods, such as fruit, vegetables, whole grains, and other plant-based foods, is associated with reduced risk of developing various CDL. Further analyses have repeatedly revealed associations between particular phytochemicals and reduced risk of a variety of CDL. These findings make it tempting to draw the conclusion that specific phytochemicals help prevent CDL. But it is important to recognize that epidemiology shows "association not causation". A major factor here is confounding as explained in Chap. 1. Whole foods typically contain not only a wide range of phytochemicals but also various micronutrients such as potassium, magnesium, vitamin C, and folate, as well as dietary fiber. This makes it extremely challenging to disentangle the effects of phytochemicals from nutrients and to prove that an association is truly a cause-and-effect-relationship.

Randomized controlled trials (RCTs) of bioactive compounds are not always consistent with findings from epidemiological studies. The following example illustrates one way this can occur. Let us suppose that a cohort study has generated findings that indicate a protective association between a phytochemical and risk of a particular disease. By contrast, an RCT failed to confirm this. In this example, the positive findings in the cohort study may be the result of substances that are present in the same foods as the phytochemical. This is an example of confounding. In this example, the negative findings of the RCT are a reflection of the low risk of confounding and therefore strongly suggest that the phytochemical does not prevent the disease.

But there are other possible explanations for inconsistencies between findings from epidemiological studies and those from RCTs. These include the dose of the phytochemicals used in RCTs, loss of bioactivity, and possible additive or synergistic effects with other substances in the food [1]. Of particular importance are the age, habitual diet, and medical history of the subjects. The one clear conclusion from this discussion is that we must exercise caution when interpreting the results of research studies, especially results that purport to show that a phytochemical lowers the risk of a particular disease. The most reliable results are those where the evidence that a phytochemical is protective against a particular disease is based on both epidemiological evidence and RCTs and where studies have been carried out by several research groups working in different countries.

This chapter reviews phytochemicals from dietary and supplemental sources and highlights the evidence regarding their relationships with human health.

Phytochemical Classifications, Food Sources, and State of the Evidence

Phytochemicals vary in their structure, distribution, relative ratios, and functions in plants. Many have been isolated and investigated to determine their actions in relation to their actions in the body and human health (Fig. 7.1). While there is no established system of categorization for phytochemicals, Table 7.1 outlines common categories, individual examples, and dietary sources.

Carotenoids

Carotenoids are richly colored substances that are the sources of the yellow, orange, and red pigments of many fruits and vegetables. α-Carotene, β-carotene, lutein, and lycopene are among the most common dietary types. α- and β-Carotene are provitamin A carotenoids, meaning they can be converted by the body to retinol. They play important roles in plant photoprotection which is related to their antioxidant activity

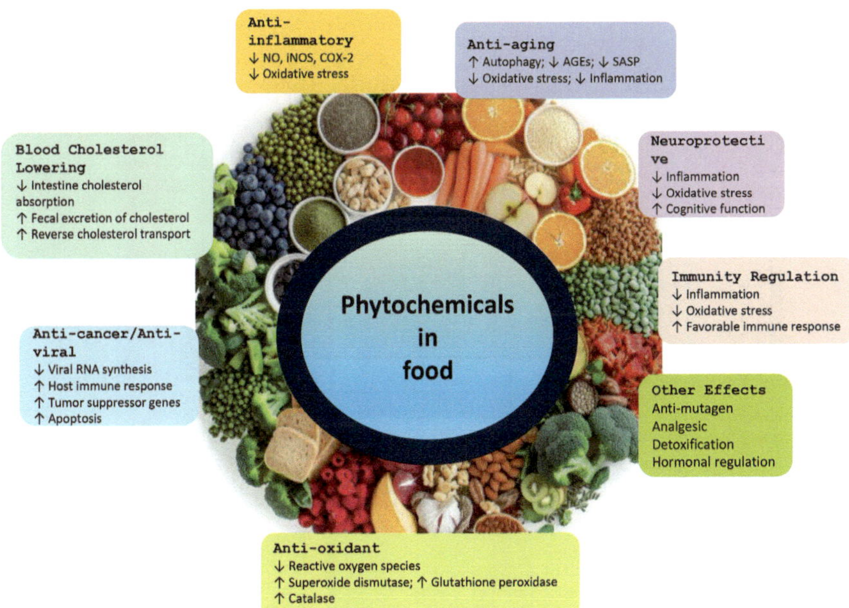

Fig. 7.1 Potential mechanisms of action in food phytochemicals. AGE advanced glycation end product, COX cyclooxygenase, iNOS inducible nitric oxide synthase, NO nitric oxide, SASP senescence-associated secretory phenotype. (Adapted from Yang and Ling, 2025 [2])

Table 1 Phytochemical categories, classification, biologic activities, and food sources

Subcategories	Classification—examples	Food sources
Carotenoids	α-Carotene β-Carotene	Apricots, carrots, sweet potatoes, pumpkin, winter squash, papaya, mango, cantaloupe
	Lutein	Dark green leafy vegetables, brightly colored fruits/vegetables
	Lycopene	Tomatoes, papaya, pink grapefruit, pink guava, watermelons
Chlorophyll	Chlorophyll a Chlorophyll b	Dark green, leafy vegetables, green foods (broccoli, green beans, parsley, asparagus, wheatgrass)
Lectins	Agglutinins Concanavalin A	Whole grains, raw legumes (jack beans, lentils, peas, soybeans, peanuts); wheat germ
Organic acids	Citric	Citrus fruit
	Oxalic	Spinach, chickpeas
Organosulfur compounds	Allylic sulfur compounds	Chives, onions, garlic, leek
	Indoles Glucosinolates	Broccoli, cauliflower, cabbage, Brussels sprouts, kale, bok choy, radishes
Nitrogen-containing compounds	Caffeine	Cocoa, coffee, tea
	Theobromine	
Capsaicinoids	Capsaicin	Chili peppers
Glucosides	Steviol glucosides	Stevia
	Cyanogenic glucosides	Flaxseed, cassava, stone and pome fruits
Phenolics: Flavonoids		
Anthocyanins		Blueberries, blackberries, cherries, plums, purple grapes
Flavanols	Catechin	Berries, apples, grapes, onions, tea, leafy greens
Flavones	Apigenin Luteolin	Celery, peppermint, thyme, parsley, buckwheat, curry leaves

Flavonols	Quercetin Kaempferol	Apples, berries, grapes, kale, onions, green and black teas
Flavanones	Hesperetin	Citrus fruits, tomatoes
Isoflavones	Glycitein Daidzein Genistein	Soybeans, legumes
Phenolics: Nonflavonoids		
Lignans		
Phenolic acids	Hydroxybenzoic acid derivatives	Apples, artichoke, barley, berries, eggplant, grapes, oranges, pears, plums, coffee, tea, green leafy vegetables, herbs (e.g., oregano, rosemary), spices
	Hydroxycinnamic acid	
Stilbenes	Resveratrol	Blueberries, cranberries, grapes, peanuts
Tannins	Condensed tannins	Grapes, sorghum, green tea
	Hydrolyzable tannins	Berries, chestnuts, carob, nuts
Phytosterols	Campesterol	Unrefined corn, sunflower, soybean oils; nuts; seeds, grains such as wheat germ, bananas, passion fruit, cauliflower, Brussels sprouts
	ß-Sitosterol	
	Stigmasterol	

in human health [3]. Carotenoids can react with free radicals and can become free radicals themselves. In sufficient concentrations, carotenoids can prevent lipid oxidation and related oxidative stress. Research about dietary carotenoids suggests they have potential role in the prevention of cancers, certain eye diseases, cardiovascular diseases (CVDs), and cognitive decline.

Cancer

A review of meta-analyses that considered multiple health outcomes reported that intake of carrots (which is rich in β-carotene) and carotene is associated with lower risk of several types of cancer [4]. This review also reported that carotene intake is associated with lower risk of fracture, cataracts, and Alzheimer's disease. Serum carotene is reported to be inversely associated with all-cause mortality, breast cancer, and lung cancer. Some evidence suggests that intake of lycopene and of tomatoes (a rich source) is associated with a reduced risk of prostate cancer [5]. In contrast to these positive studies, some RCTs reported an increased risk of lung cancer after β-carotene supplementation. This has led the US Preventive Services Task Force to discourage use of this supplement [6].

Eye Diseases

Lutein and zeaxanthin are found in the retina. They are efficient absorbers of blue light and may help protect against light-induced oxidative damage. The results of cohort studies suggest that high intakes of foods rich in these carotenoids reduce the likelihood of cataract development [7].

Metabolic-Associated Diseases

There is strong evidence that carotenoids improve adiposity and lipid profiles [6]. A meta-analysis reported 12–18% lower risk of coronary heart disease and stroke in individuals in the highest versus lowest tertile of blood lutein concentration [8]. Lower serum concentrations of various carotenoids were associated with higher risk of all-cause and cardiovascular mortality in US adults with metabolic (dysfunction)-associated fatty liver disease (MAFLD) [9].

Cognitive Function

Carotenoids such as lutein and zeaxanthin can cross the blood-brain barrier. A meta-analysis of observational studies reported that individuals with dementia had lower blood levels of several carotenoids compared to controls suggesting that lower blood carotenoid levels may be a risk factor for dementia and mild cognitive impairment [10]. Supplementation with lutein and zeaxanthin may improve cognitive performance [11], however further investigations are needed to confirm this.

Nitrogen-Containing Compounds

Major classes of these compounds include the alkaloids. These are a structurally diverse group which include tryptophan-derived indole alkaloids (e.g., ergotin) and purine alkaloids (e.g., caffeine, theobromine). They are associated with beneficial health effects, such as quinine for antimalaria, while some can be toxic. Capsaicin, one of the active ingredients in chili peppers, has been reported to have anticarcinogenic, antimicrobial, antidiabetic, hypolipidemic, and antiobesity effects, but epidemiological evidence has been inconclusive [12]. Caffeine and theobromine show stimulant activities, and their therapeutic efficiencies are under study in pain management and anticancer therapies [13]. Avenanthramides are plant alkaloids found primarily in oats that may help to prevent atherosclerosis [14]. However, as with many observational studies of the association between intake of phytochemicals and reduced risk of disease, we cannot draw firm conclusions, mainly because of the possibility of confounding.

Glucosinolates are a class of substances derived from amino acids that include sulfur. Cruciferous vegetables are major sources and evidence suggests that intake of these foods is associated with beneficial effects in gastric, lung, and endometrial cancer as well as all-cause mortality [15]. More research is needed on individual glucosinolates in relation to cancer.

Phenolics

Phenolics are a diverse group of plant-based molecules with a chemical structure that contains at least one phenol unit. Polyphenols are a subclass and are the major type of phenolics. Polyphenols are divided into two groups: flavonoids and nonflavonoids.

Flavonoids

Of all the different types of phytochemicals it is this group of polyphenols that has the strongest supporting evidence that they enhance health and reduce risk of a variety of CDL. This was clearly demonstrated in a cohort study of 86,400 American men and women aged over 60. Total intake of flavonoids manifested a clear protective association with a 12% lower risk of both impaired physical function and poor mental health [16]. The dominant foods supplying flavonoids to the subjects were tea, apples, oranges, grapefruits, blueberries, strawberries, and red wine.

Flavonoids are subdivided into several groups including anthocyanins, flavanols, flavonols, flavones, flavanones, and isoflavones.

- Anthocyanins are associated with multiple health benefits. These include improvements in blood lipids, bone health, and reduced risk of CVDs, hypertension, type 2 diabetes, certain cancers, cognitive decline, metabolic syndrome, and obesity [17, 18]. Anthocyanins have antioxidant, anti-inflammatory, and metabolic regulatory properties which are likely to be at least partly responsible for many of these positive effects on health.
- Flavanols include catechins of which epigallocatechin (EGCG) has the most biological activity. EGCG is found in green and black tea. Cohort studies have demonstrated that tea intake has an inverse association with risk of CVD [19] and

cognitive decline [20]. Strong evidence indicates that EGCG is the component of tea responsible for this benefit. In addition, catechins have been reported to have several other beneficial properties including antioxidant and anti-inflammatory activity [21].

- The flavonols quercetin and kaempferol and the flavones luteolin and apigenin have been reported to have cardioprotective effects [22]. Research findings suggest that the impact of quercetin on blood pressure and CVD risk is limited [23]. Epidemiological studies and some clinical trials suggest that a daily intake of ≥1.5 mg/day of kaempferol is associated with lower risk of coronary disease.
- Flavanones have been reported to have antioxidant, anti-inflammatory, anticancer, and antidiabetic properties, but these benefits need to be verified in human trials [24].
- Isoflavones are largely known as phytoestrogens. Daidzein and genistein are isoflavones that are being studied for their chemotherapeutic potential for invasive cancer [25]. Isoflavones combined with vitamin D have been reported to have positive synergistic effects in relation to bone mineral density [26]. Isoflavones can also bind to estrogen receptors. In a meta-analysis of observational studies it was reported that soy isoflavones were associated with a 26% reduced risk of breast cancer recurrence, particularly among postmenopausal and estrogen receptor-positive women [27]. Soy protein and products were inversely associated with cancer-specific mortality for estrogen receptor-positive disease.

Non-flavonoids

Non-flavonoids are distinct phenolic compounds and are divided into several groups. Lignans, which possess a steroid-like chemical structure, are of investigative interest. Flaxseeds are among the richest sources of lignan precursors in the human diet but are also good sources of nutrients and phytochemicals with cardioprotective effects, such as α-linolenic acid and fiber. While most research on phytoestrogen-rich diets has focused on soy isoflavones [28], lignans are the principal source of dietary phytoestrogens in the typical Western diet. Lignans are associated with lower risk of CVD, menopausal symptoms, and osteoporosis as well as breast and colon cancer.

Phenolic acids are found in many plants and their content is particularly high in dried fruit. Of their two subclasses, hydroxybenzoic and hydroxycinnamic acid, the latter is more widely studied. Hydroxycinnamic acid, which interacts with the gut microbiota, may have positive effects on colorectal cancer, inflammatory bowel diseases, mental-cognitive impairments, nonalcoholic liver disease, and obesity [29]. Chlorogenic acid is a derivative of hydroxycinnamic acid has attracted much attention. It reportedly has wide-ranging beneficial actions including antioxidant, anti-inflammatory, anticancer, antibacterial, hepatoprotective, and neuroprotective effects [30]. Studies indicate that it may play a significant role in the prevention and treatment of many chronic diseases, including type 2 diabetes, obesity, hypertension, dyslipidemia, and cardiovascular diseases. However, the substance has a relatively low bioavailability which may limit its beneficial action on health. Major sources include coffee, tea, fruits, and vegetables.

Stilbenes are another group of phenolic compounds with diverse biological activities. Resveratrol is the most studied stilbene. Based on more than 200 RCTs across several health outcomes, including cancer, menopause symptoms, diabetes, metabolic syndrome, and CVD, a picture emerges that resveratrol consistently reduces inflammatory markers and improves components of dysregulated metabolism such as elevated triglycerides [31, 32].

The final group of phenolic compounds to be considered are tannins. They are broadly categorized into hydrolyzable and condensed tannins. Tannins have been associated with a reduced risk of CVD, cancer, and diabetes [33]. Similar to other antinutritional components, tannins that are present in legume seeds can bind to minerals and reduce their bioavailability.

Curcumin

Curcumin is another type of phenolic but is classified separately from the above phenolics. It is found in the turmeric plant. It has been investigated regarding its potential beneficial effects in the therapy of CVDs, cancers, and systemic inflammation. A meta-analysis based on 103 RCTs reported clear evidence that turmeric improves blood sugar, C-reactive protein, high-density lipoprotein cholesterol, and weight [34]. Some evidence suggests that turmeric extract and curcumin supplements may be beneficial for musculoskeletal health [35]. A systematic review that evaluated 15 RCTs saw generally positive evidence that curcumin has diverse therapeutic effects in combating age-related disorders. In particular, it improves cognitive function and reduces neurodegeneration in the elderly persons [36]. Oral supplementation with curcumin is generally regarded as safe.

Phytosterols

Phytosterols are structurally similar to cholesterol. They are added to some brands of margarines. They decrease cholesterol absorption, reduce total cholesterol and LDL-cholesterol, and may therefore furnish some protection against heart disease [37].

Organosulfur Compounds

As the name suggests, organosulfur-containing compounds (OSCs) include sulfur in their structure. They are found in plant foods such as garlic, onions, legumes, and cruciferous vegetables such as cabbage. OSCs are highly reactive. Of the different food-based OSCs, garlic has been the most widely studied with systematic reviews reporting beneficial effects on blood pressure, waist circumference, BMI, and blood lipids [38]. Other evidence indicates that the benefits of garlic include antioxidant, hypoglycemic, anti-inflammatory, anticancer, antimicrobial, and hepatoprotective activities [39]. Research studies suggest that consuming foods that are high in sulfur has beneficial effects on brain function [40].

Lectins

Epidemiological studies have reported that a lectin-rich diet is associated with lower risk of CVD, type 2 diabetes, cancer, and mortality [41]. Research findings also suggest that lectins have other health benefits including antimicrobial, antifungal, and antiviral activities [42]. However, lectins may also have some potentially harmful effects. They may trigger the production of particular antibodies which can provoke food allergies. Lectins may be considered as antinutrient phytochemicals and contribute to shortage of essential nutrients, particularly in vulnerable individuals. Applying different conventional processing or cooking techniques can reduce the lectin content of food.

Phytochemicals in Foods and Antagonistic Effects

While the focus has been on the health benefits of phytochemicals, it is also important to recognize that some have potential negative effects or antagonistic effects where one phytochemical may reduce or counteract the biological activity of another, decrease its efficacy, or enhance toxicity (Fig. 7.2) [42]. Antagonism can be dependent on a variety of factors such as the specific chemical properties and concentrations of the phytochemicals. Additional research is needed to provide knowledge that can leverage additive and synergistic effects and minimize or avoid antagonistic effects in daily diets or phytochemical-based interventions.

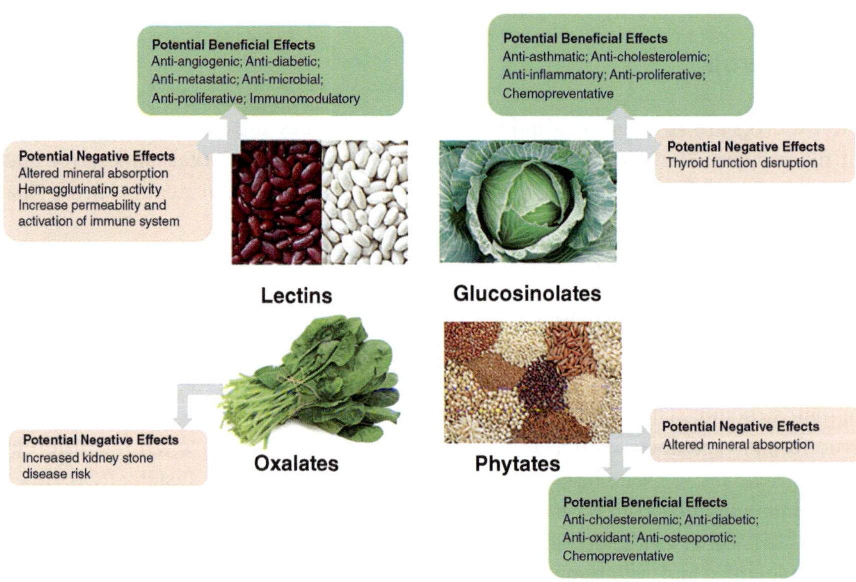

Fig. 7.2 Potential beneficial and negative effects of select phytochemicals. (Adapted from López-Moreno [42])

Phytochemicals in Foods: Considerations

To advance understanding about the role of phytochemicals in food, a number of factors need to be considered. It remains largely unknown whether the beneficial effects of consuming plant-based foods are due to specific nutrients or phytochemicals. Continued applications in nutrigenomics and metabolomics will deepen our understanding of the impact of phytochemicals on health. Future research also needs to consider the dose-response relationship of phytochemicals [1]. For example, the Chinese Nutrition Society established specific proposed levels (SPL) for phytochemicals in their latest *Dietary Reference Intakes*. The SPL refers to the recommended level of intake that promotes health and decreases risk of chronic diseases. While the SPL are mainly based on cohort studies and some RCTs, the values will become more relevant as phytochemistry research progresses.

Future research about phytochemicals needs to include advancements in molecular research as well as providing better means of quantitative measurement. Furthermore, there needs to be recognition of the ever-changing molecular mechanisms by organisms in growth, development, metabolism, and movement [1]. Research using molecular cloning, gene chip technology, and single-molecule techniques will help explain the different biological effects in response to dietary phytochemicals. Current food and nutrient databases and dietary data collection methods provide information about the essential macro- and micronutrients in foods but lack data on phytochemicals. Resolving issues of accurately measuring phytochemicals or their specific metabolites in the body will advance knowledge that can support evidence-based dietary guidelines for global health.

Investigations about the effects of phytochemicals on human health need to consider the intestinal microecology and outcome measures. How microbiome alterations serve as moderators or mediators between phytochemicals and health outcomes needs further exploration. Most observational studies have focused on the dietary phytochemical intake and terminal outcomes such as morbidity or mortality rather than the intermediate processes (e.g., blood lipid profiles, inflammation). Strengthening population and experimental research will help to better understand the potential benefits of phytochemicals.

Conclusion

Phytochemicals represent a vital link between plant-based foods and human health. Hundreds of research studies in recent years have firmly established the critical importance of these substances. By incorporating a diverse array of fruits, vegetables, whole grains, legumes, nuts, seeds, and teas into the diet, people can harness the health benefits of these bioactive compounds. Continued research that considers factors such as additive and synergistic actions, interactions with the gut microbiome, and genotyping of participants promises to uncover even greater therapeutic potential in phytochemicals for preventing and managing disease.

References

1. Blumfield M, Mayr H, De Vlieger N, Abbott K, Starck C, Fayet-Moore F, et al. Should we 'Eat a Rainbow'? An umbrella review of the health effects of colorful bioactive pigments in fruits and vegetables. Molecules. 2022;27:4061.
2. Yang Y, Ling W. Health benefits and future research of phytochemicals: a literature review. J Nutr. 2025;155:87–101.
3. Bin-Jumah MN, Nadeem MS, Gilani SJ, Mubeen B, Ullah I, Alzarea SI, et al. Lycopene: a natural arsenal in the war against oxidative stress and cardiovascular diseases. Antioxidants. 2022;2022(11):232.
4. Yi X, Li J, Liao D, Peng G, Zheng X, Xu H, et al. Carrot and carotene and multiple health outcomes: an umbrella review of the evidence. J Sci Food Agric. 2023;103:2251–61.
5. Sadeghian M, Asadi M, Rahmani S, Sadeghi N, Hosseini SA, Zare JA. Lycopene does not affect prostate-specific antigen in men with non-metastatic prostate cancer: a systematic review and meta-analysis of randomized controlled trials. Nutr Cancer. 2021;73:2796–807.
6. Kordiak J, Bielec F, Jabłoński S, Pastuszak-Lewandoska D. Role of beta-carotene in lung cancer primary chemoprevention: a systematic review with meta-analysis and meta-regression. Nutrients. 2022;14:1361.
7. Mrowicka M, Mrowicki J, Kucharska E, Majsterek I. Lutein and zeaxanthin and their roles in age-related macular degeneration-neurodegenerative disease. Nutrients. 2022;14:827.
8. Leermakers ET, Darweesh SK, Baena CP, Moreira EM, Melo van Lent D, Tielemans MJ, et al. The effects of lutein on cardiometabolic health across the life course: a systematic review and meta-analysis. Am J Clin Nutr. 2016;103:481–94.
9. Lin B, Liu Z, Li D, Zhang T, Yu C. Associations of serum carotenoids with all-cause and cardiovascular mortality in adults with MAFLD. Nutr Metab Cardiovasc Dis. 2024;34:2315–24.
10. Wang L, Zhao T, Zhu X, Jiang Q. Low blood carotenoid status in dementia and mild cognitive impairment: a systematic review and meta-analysis. BMC Geriatr. 2023;23:195.
11. Stringham NT, Holmes PV, Stringham JM. Effects of macular xanthophyll supplementation on brain-derived neurotrophic factor, pro-inflammatory cytokines, and cognitive performance. Physiol Behav. 2019;211:112650.
12. Ao Z, Huang Z, Liu H. Spicy food and chili peppers and multiple health outcomes: umbrella review. Mol Nutr Food Res. 2022;66:e2200167.
13. Kamiloglu SE, Capanoglu E, Jafari SM. An overview of food bioactive compounds and their health-promoting features. In: Jafari SM, Capanoglu E, editors. Retention of bioactives in food processing. Cham: Springer; 2022. p. 3–36.
14. Sang S, Chu Y. Whole grain oats, more than just a fiber: role of unique phytochemicals. Mol Nutr Food Res. 2017;61:1770074.
15. Li YZ, Yang ZY, Gong TT, Liu YS, Liu FH, Wen ZY, et al. Cruciferous vegetable consumption and multiple health outcomes: an umbrella review of 41 systematic reviews and meta-analyses of 303 observational studies. Food Funct. 2022;13:4247–59.
16. Bondonno NP, Liu YL, Grodstein F, Rimm EB, Cassidy A. Associations between flavonoid-rich food and flavonoid intakes and incident unhealthy aging outcomes in older United States males and females. Am J Clin Nutr. 2025;121:972–85.
17. Ma X, Li B, Liu Y, Guo X. An inverted U shaped association between high-sensitivity C-reactive protein and the albumin ratio and hepatic steatosis and liver fibrosis: a population-based study. Front Nutr. 2025;12:1534200.
18. Panchal SK, John OD, Mathai ML, Brown L. Anthocyanins in chronic diseases: the power of purple. Nutrients. 2022;14:2161.
19. Bhandari B, Zeng L, Grafenauer S, Schutte AE, Xu X. Long-term consumption of 6 different beverages and cardiovascular disease-related mortality: a systematic review and meta-analysis of prospective cohort studies. Curr Dev Nutr. 2024;8:102095.
20. Zhu Y, Hu CX, Liu X, Zhu RX, Wang BQ. Moderate coffee or tea consumption decreased the risk of cognitive disorders: an updated dose-response meta-analysis. Nutr Rev. 2024;82:738–48.

21. Ferrari E, Naponelli V. Catechins and human health: breakthroughs from clinical trials. Molecules. 2025;30:3128.
22. Chagas MDSS, Behrens MD, Moragas-Tellis CJ, Penedo GXM, Silva AR, Gonçalves-de-Albuquerque CF. Flavonols and flavones as potential anti-inflammatory, antioxidant, and antibacterial compounds. Oxidative Med Cell Longev. 2022;2022:9966750.
23. Dabeek WM, Marra MV. Dietary quercetin and kaempferol: bioavailability and potential cardiovascular-related bioactivity in humans. Nutrients. 2019;11:2288.
24. Azhar S, Sabahat R, Sajjad R, Nadeem F, Amjad A, Hafeez N, et al. Effect of citrus flavanones on diabetes: a systematic review. Curr Diabetes Rev. 2023;19:e070722206679.
25. Cayetano-Salazar L, Olea-Flores M, Zuñiga-Eulogio MD, Weinstein-Oppenheimer C, Fernández-Tilapa G, Mendoza-Catalán MA, et al. Natural isoflavonoids in invasive cancer therapy: from bench to bedside. Phytother Res. 2021;35:4092–110.
26. Miedziaszczyk M, Maciejewski A, Idasiak-Piechocka I, Karczewski M, Lacka K. Effects of isoflavonoid and vitamin D synergism on bone mineral density-a systematic and critical review. Nutrients. 2023;15:5014.
27. van Die MD, Bone KM, Visvanathan K, Kyrø C, Aune D, Ee C, et al. Phytonutrients and outcomes following breast cancer: a systematic review and meta-analysis of observational studies. JNCI Cancer Spectr. 2024;8:pkad104.
28. Rodríguez-García C, Sánchez-Quesada C, Toledo E, Delgado-Rodríguez M, Gaforio JJ. Naturally lignan-rich foods: a dietary tool for health promotion? Molecules. 2019;24:917.
29. Leonard W, Zhang P, Ying D, Fang Z. Hydroxycinnamic acids on gut microbiota and health. Compr Rev Food Sci Food Saf. 2021;20:710–37.
30. Zalewska K, Kulawik M, Gierszewska J, Gramala Z, Kalus O, Karpiński M, et al. Chlorogenic acid's role in metabolic health: mechanisms and therapeutic potential. Nutrients. 2025;17:3303.
31. Shao Y, Shi J. Anti-inflammatory mechanism of resveratrol's triglyceride-lowering effect in hyperlipidemia: a meta-analysis integrated network pharmacology and molecular dynamics simulation. Clin Exp Med. 2025;25:262.
32. Brown K, Theofanous D, Britton RG, Aburido G, Pepper C, Sri Undru S, et al. Resveratrol for the management of human health: how far have we come? A systematic review of resveratrol clinical trials to highlight gaps and opportunities. Int J Mol Sci. 2024;25:747.
33. Oliveira I, Vilela A, Gonçalves B. A comprehensive review of bioactive tannins in foods and beverages: functional properties, health benefits, and sensory qualities. Molecules. 2025;30:800.
34. Jafari A, Abbastabar M, Alaghi A, Heshmati J, Crowe FL, Sepidarkish M. Curcumin on human health: a comprehensive systematic review and meta-analysis of 103 randomized controlled trials. Phytother Res. 2024;38:6048–61.
35. Doyle L, Desomayanandam P, Bhuvanendran A, Thanawala S, Shah R, Somepalli V, et al. Safety and efficacy of turmeric (Curcuma longa) extract and curcumin supplements in musculoskeletal health: a systematic review and meta-analysis. Altern Ther Health Med. 2023;29:12–24.
36. Nunes YC, Mendes NM, Pereira de Lima E, Chehadi AC, Lamas CB, Haber JFS, et al. Curcumin: a golden approach to healthy aging: a systematic review of the evidence. Nutrients. 2024;16:2721.
37. Liu B, Chen K, Chen X, Wang J, Shu G, Ping Z, et al. Health outcomes associated with phytosterols: an umbrella review of systematic reviews and meta-analyses of randomized controlled trials. Phytomedicine. 2024;122:155151.
38. Imaizumi VM, Laurindo LF, Manzan B, Guiguer EL, Oshiiwa M, Otoboni AMMB, et al. Garlic: a systematic review of the effects on cardiovascular diseases. Crit Rev Food Sci Nutr. 2023;63:6797–819.
39. Tudu CK, Dutta T, Ghorai M, Biswas P, Samanta D, Oleksak P, et al. Traditional uses, phytochemistry, pharmacology and toxicology of garlic (*Allium sativum*), a storehouse of diverse phytochemicals: a review of research from the last decade focusing on health and nutritional implications. Front Nutr. 2022;9:949554.

40. Rana A, Katiyar A, Arun A, Berrios JN, Kumar G. Natural sulfur compounds in mental health and neurological disorders: insights from observational and intervention studies. Front Nutr. 2025;12:1534000.
41. Konozy EHE, Osman MEM. From inflammation to immune regulation: the dual nature of dietary lectins in health and disease. Heliyon. 2024;10:e39471.
42. López-Moreno M, Garcés-Rimón M, Miguel M. Antinutrients: lectins, goitrogens, phytates and oxalates, friends or foe? J Funct Foods. 2022;89:104938.

Food Synergy: A Paradigm Shift in Nutrition Science

8

David R. Jacobs Jr and Norman J. Temple

Abstract

- A major focus of nutrition science has traditionally centered on identifying the various macronutrients, vitamins, and minerals and then investigating their mode of action.
- The concept of food synergy challenges this strategy for understanding nutrition science.
- The argument is presented that many associations between diet and risk of disease are best understood by looking at foods and dietary patterns as a whole and not merely as a collection of individual nutrients and other bioactive substances.
- The following argument provides additional support for the concept of food synergy. Because of the limitations of epidemiology, it is extremely difficult in most cases to identify the substances in food that account for protection against disease. This is especially the case with phytochemical-rich plant foods, including fruit, vegetables, nuts, legumes, and whole-grain cereal foods.

Most research that has investigated the relationship between diet and disease historically has focused on studying single substances: macronutrients, micronutrients, as well as the many other bioactive substances present in food, either beneficial or

D. R. Jacobs Jr
Division of Epidemiology and Community Health, School of Public Health, University of Minnesota, Minneapolis, MN, USA
e-mail: Jacobs@epi.umn.edu

N. J. Temple (✉)
Centre for Science, Athabasca University, Athabasca, AB, Canada
e-mail: normant@athabascau.ca

N. J. Temple, T. Wilson (eds.), *Pocket Primer for Nutritional Health*,
https://doi.org/10.1007/978-3-032-25402-3_8

harmful. Here we argue the case for turning our attention to food as a whole and to dietary patterns. The constituents of foods and of dietary patterns act in concert to influence health. This concept, known as food synergy, is defined as additive or more than additive influences of foods and food constituents on health. It is a powerful tool that helps explain many nutrition-related diseases and how best to prevent and treat them. Many ideas in this chapter were stated some years ago by one of us (DJ) [1–5]. Other authors have endorsed this concept [6–8].

The Concept of Nutrient Deficiency Diseases

Up until the 1950s, a major focus of nutrition science centered on identifying the various vitamins and minerals and then discovering their mode of action [7]. The underlying reasoning is as follows:

1. There is a simple cause-and-effect relationship between deficiency of a nutrient and the associated disease.
2. Each nutrient deficiency disease can be explained in terms of the role played by that nutrient, especially in the areas of biochemistry and physiology.
3. The nutrient deficiency can be prevented (and often reversed) by giving that nutrient in a pure form.

Classic examples are vitamin C in relation to scurvy and iron in relation to anemia. This concept is still very much alive and is seen in the vitamin and mineral chapters of every nutrition textbook. The concept can also be applied to protein and essential fats.

In recent years, the concept has shown its continuing value. For example, research has demonstrated that supplementary folic acid (a form of folate) is protective against neural tube defects (NTD), a group of congenital disorders that include spina bifida [9]. It appears that a low maternal intake of folate creates a deficiency condition in the fetus that hinders normal development of the nervous system, thereby allowing the condition to emerge [10]. As a result of this discovery, mandatory addition of folic acid to refined grain products started in 1998 in the USA and Canada.

The relationship between single substances and disease risk extends well beyond prevention by micronutrients; there are many other bioactive substances in food, either beneficial or harmful. As an example, the great majority of the population consume a high intake of sodium (as salt). This plays an important role in the causation of hypertension and cardiovascular disease (CVD) (Chap. 3). *Trans*-fatty acids are another example. These fats adversely affect multiple cardiovascular risk factors and increase the risk of coronary heart disease (CHD) (Chap. 3).

But in many cases we find that this reductionist approach to nutrition has not provided accurate information regarding which aspects of diet have a cause-and-effect relationship with disease risk. This is best demonstrated by studies in which observational studies suggested that particular nutrients are associated with reduced risk of particular diseases. These nutrients were then used in higher doses as supplements in clinical trials. But the purified nutrients did not work as predicted according to reductionist logic. Beta-carotene is a well-known example of this [11].

Food Synergy: An Alternative Paradigm

The Emergence of the Concept of Food Synergy

Based on the above reasoning, there is a compelling case that to properly explain the many associations between diet and risk of disease, we should view food as a whole and not merely as a collection of nutrients and other bioactive substances. This concept has emerged during the present century. In a nutshell—figuratively (and literally in the case of nuts)—food synergy has provided an explanation based on an impressive weight of evidence for many nutrition-related diseases and how best to prevent and treat them. This represents a paradigm shift in our understanding of nutrition science.

Strong support for food synergy comes from examining complex dietary patterns in relation to disease risk. The following examples illustrate this.

The Mediterranean Diet

The Mediterranean diet and its effects on health has attracted enormous interest. The diet is discussed in some detail in Chap. 5. While this diet varies from country to country around the Mediterranean, major features include a relatively high intake of vegetables, fruit, legumes, nuts, fish, cereals, and olive oil. Conversely, the diet is typically low in meat, especially red meat, such as beef and pork, and processed meat.

Strong evidence demonstrates that consumption of the diet reduces the risk of cardiovascular disease. This was demonstrated in the large, long-term PREDIMED randomized controlled trial [12] and in another randomized trial [13]. Further confirmation came from a systematic review and meta-analysis of observational studies [14].

The Mediterranean diet has a complex nutritional composition. It is rich in phytochemicals but low in saturated fat, heme iron, and many other substances found in meat. It appears highly likely that multiple dietary components and multiple pathways are at work. It can therefore be argued that this diet–disease association provides strong support for the food synergy concept.

Healthy and Unhealthy Dietary Patterns

The Mediterranean diet is just one example of a healthy dietary pattern. Several others have been proposed. One is the Alternate Healthy Eating Index, as revised in 2010 [15]. The diet is based on foods that cohort studies show are associated with a reduced risk of various chronic diseases, such as CVD and cancer. Another is the Planetary Health Diet proposed by the EAT-Lancet Commission on "Healthy Diets from Sustainable Food Systems" (EAT-Lancet) [16]. This diet is designed to be both healthy and sustainable for the planet. A third example is the DASH Diet. Key features are a generous intake of fruit, vegetables, and low-fat dairy products, combined with a reduced intake of meat and therefore of saturated fat. It was developed as a treatment for hypertension and has proven effective (Chap. 5). Cohort studies have provided compelling evidence that all three of these diets are associated with improved health and a reduced risk of chronic diseases [17, 18].

Just as every movie with a hero also needs a villain, so a study of healthy dietary patterns needs an unhealthy one. That role is played by the "Western" pattern. Such a diet is high in red meat, processed meat, refined cereals, and foods with a high sugar content. This diet is similar to the reference diet eaten in cohort studies and which have demonstrated the health benefits of the previous diets.

In the past, researchers would attempt to explain the above findings in terms of individual substances. Healthy diets, for example, generally have a high content of vitamin C, folate, magnesium, potassium, and dietary fiber but a low content of saturated fat and sugar. But this comparison fails to properly explain a far more complex story. Of particular importance, a feature of the typical Western diet is a high content of ultra-processed foods. These foods typically have a high energy density and various other characteristics which trick the appetite and lead people to eat an excessive amount of food energy (Chap. 4). By contrast, healthy diets are usually rich in phytochemicals. There are thousands of these substances. We are only beginning to understand their relationship with health and risk of disease.

It seems very unlikely that we will ever be able to fully explain which substances in foods are associated with each chronic disease. There is strong evidence in support of this conclusion. First, and most obviously, there are a large number of individual substances present in food. Explaining which combination causes or prevents each disease means decoding a vast permutation of possibilities. But there is an additional and perhaps even greater challenge to overcome. The individual substances in foods are almost certainly acting in concert (i.e., food synergy), not independently of each other. This adds a whole layer of great complexity. Based on this reasoning we must conclude that the relationship between diet and disease should be viewed, in the large majority of cases, in terms of foods and dietary patterns. This conclusion reinforces the arguments supporting the case for food synergy that were made earlier.

Red Meat, Processed Meat, and Health

We now look at food synergy from another perspective by moving from the big picture (dietary patterns) to the smaller picture (individual foods). The focus here is red and processed meat.

There has been much interest regarding the relationship between meat consumption and health. Vegetarian diets have been advocated in some quarters for many decades as a healthier alternative to a meat-based diet. Cohort studies have provided solid evidence that red and processed meat are associated with an increased risk of CVD and all-cause mortality [19, 20]. This points to the health benefits of a reduced intake of red and processed meat.

There are several possible substances that might explain these results, including saturated fat, iron, and various amino acids, and an absence of phytochemicals. Many nutritional factors are probably involved in the connection between meat and risk of diverse diseases. Likewise, there are many additives in processed meat that might harm health. Accordingly, consumption of red and processed should best be viewed from the perspective of food synergy.

Essentially the same argument can be made for the association between intake of fruit, vegetables, and whole grain cereals and risk of various chronic diseases (except, of course, that these foods manifest a protective association).

Food Synergy and Disease: A Summary

In each of the above cases, we see strong evidence that the relationship between diet and disease risk is best explained by focusing on foods rather than single substances present in food. This applies to both prevention and treatment. It also applies both to dietary patterns and to single food groups such as fruit and meat. These conclusions are a reflection of the great complexity of food and dietary patterns, the thousands of different substances present, and the many pathways that connect food with the etiology of disease. As a result, the impact of dietary patterns and of single food groups on disease risk is the result of highly complex interactions of many different substances.

Food Synergy and the Limitations of Epidemiology

The evidence considered above supports the case for food synergy. There is a separate line of argument that adds additional support for the concept. Nutrition research methods have limited power to identify which nutrients or other bioactive substances in a complex food are likely to be responsible for an association (positive or negative) with the risk of particular diseases. The reasons for this were explained in Chap. 1. The major problem is that nutrients and other bioactive substances are not distributed randomly in foods. Instead, they are commonly associated with each other. As a result, focusing on one substance causes confounding duc to the presence of many other substances. This problem is especially acute with the multitude of substances found in fruit and vegetables and other phytochemical-rich plant foods. We see, therefore, that the problem of confounding makes it extremely difficult to identify which nutrients or other bioactive substances deserve the credit for the health benefits of such foods as fruit, vegetables, and whole grain cereals.

One obvious way to circumvent this problem is to carry out randomized controlled trials (RCTs) on single substances. However, these are extremely costly and usually take several years. They are only appropriate, therefore, when dealing with dietary components where there is already strong supporting evidence. Before undertaking an RCT on a single substance derived from food, it is important to be clear about whether it is even possible to determine the health implications of a single nutritional substance. As well, one must consider whether the findings from that RCT would help elucidate what food people should eat.

Conclusions

Food that emanates from a living organism is a mixture of a great many constituents but is not a random mixture. Rather, the particular mixture has proven adequate through evolution for the life of that organism. To the extent that the organism has been eaten for a long time, evolution has also tested the mixture of constituents as a food for the eater.

There is a strong case for placing much more emphasis on food synergy and regarding findings for foods or dietary patterns as final answers to questions. This can include dietary patterns, such as the Mediterranean diet, or single foods, such as red meat. It is not clear whether food synergy reflects a true mathematical synergistic relationship (i.e., the whole risk or benefit is greater than the sum of the parts) or else is simply an additive effect. At minimum, though, even in the absence of mathematical synergy, foods are complex mixtures, tested by evolution, which we would not come to by constituting them de novo from individual constituents.

We have stressed that the most productive research strategy is one focused on foods and dietary patterns rather than single substances. But there are many exceptions to this rule. There is still much to be gained from research that investigates individual nutrients and bioactive substances in food and then attempts to determine their role in health and disease. This is especially valuable in cases where problems of confounding are relatively small and it is therefore possible to investigate nutrients or other substances as single variables. Sodium (salt) and vitamin D are excellent example of this.

In several cases, research on single nutrients has led to important measures that have improved public health. We see this with folate in relation to spina bifida. Other notable cases of single-nutrient solutions to health problems are iron supplementation for iron-deficiency anemia and vitamin B_{12} supplementation for the elderly. However, these instances usually occur in situations of relative deficiency.

We must stay open to the possibility of more such cases appearing. It is entirely possible that some phytochemicals will be proven to have valuable health-enhancing actions. Indeed, some evidence of this has already been documented. For example, lutein is showing promise for improving eye health [21] and anthocyanins for giving protection against type 2 diabetes, bringing about desirable changes in the blood levels of glucose and lipids, and lowering the BMI [22, 23]. The credit may belong to a single substance or to a group of closely related substances. Whether these substances would be useful as supplements in the general population is an unanswered question; or, perhaps they should be thought of as drugs.

We are sympathetic to attempts to properly understand the detailed causes of chronic diseases. However, we believe that the complexity of metabolism and pathology is such that nutrition research is a long way from being able to achieve this goal. Epidemiologic studies of nutrients are often misleading because they miss the context of the whole food and diet pattern. In other words, both epidemiologic study of nutrients and mechanistic research are inferior strategies for achieving valuable breakthroughs that lead to improvements in public health through improved diet. Despite that, mechanistic research attracts far more resources than food-based research. We conclude, therefore, that improved infrastructure for food-oriented research would be most valuable.

References

1. Messina M, Lampe JW, Birt DF, et al. Reductionism and the narrowing nutrition perspective: time for reevaluation and emphasis on food synergy. J Am Diet Assoc. 2001;101:1416–9.
2. Jacobs DR, Murtaugh MA. It's more than an apple a day: an appropriately processed plant-centered dietary pattern may be good for your health. Am J Clin Nutr. 2000;72:899–900.
3. Jacobs DR, Steffen LM. Nutrients, foods, and dietary patterns as exposures in research: a framework for food synergy. Am J Clin Nutr. 2003;78(Suppl):508S–13S.
4. Jacobs DR Jr, Tapsell LC. Food, not nutrients, is the fundamental unit in nutrition. Nutr Rev. 2007;65:439–50.
5. Jacobs DR Jr, Orlich MJ. Diet pattern and longevity: do simple rules suffice? A commentary. Am J Clin Nutr. 2014;100(Suppl 1):313S–9S.
6. Tapsell LC, Neale EP, Satija A, Hu FB. Foods, nutrients, and dietary patterns: interconnections and implications for dietary guidelines. Adv Nutr. 2016;7:445–54.
7. Mozaffarian D, Rosenberg UR. History of modern nutrition science-implications for current research, dietary guidelines, and food policy. BMJ. 2018;361:k2392.
8. Fardet A, Rock E. Perspective: reductionist nutrition research has meaning only within the framework of holistic and ethical thinking. Adv Nutr. 2018;9:655–70.
9. Wolff T, Witkop CT, Miller T, Syed SB, U.S. Preventive Services Task Force. Folic acid supplementation for the prevention of neural tube defects: an update of the evidence for the U.S. preventive services task force. Ann Intern Med. 2009;150:632–9.
10. Jacobs DR Jr, Mursu J, Meyer KA. The importance of food. Arch Pediatr Adolesc Med. 2012;166:187–8.
11. Druesne-Pecollo N, Latino-Martel P, Norat T, Barrandon E, Bertrais S, Galan P, et al. Beta-carotene supplementation and cancer risk: a systematic review and metaanalysis of randomized controlled trials. Int J Cancer. 2010;127:172–84.
12. Estruch R, Ros E, Salas-Salvadó J, et al. PREDIMED study investigators. Primary prevention of cardiovascular disease with a Mediterranean diet supplemented with extra-virgin olive oil or nuts. N Engl J Med. 2018;378:e34.

13. Delgado-Lista J, Alcala-Diaz JF, Torres-Peña JD, Quintana-Navarro GM, Fuentes F, Garcia-Rios A, et al. CORDIOPREV investigators. Long-term secondary prevention of cardiovascular disease with a Mediterranean diet and a low-fat diet (CORDIOPREV): a randomised controlled trial. Lancet. 2022;399:1876–85.
14. Rosato V, Temple NJ, La Vecchia C, Castellan G, Tavani A, Guercio V. Mediterranean diet and cardiovascular disease: a systematic review and meta-analysis of observational studies. Eur J Nutr. 2019;58:173–91.
15. Chiuve SE, Fung TT, Rexrode KM, Spiegelman D, Manson JE, Stampfer MJ, et al. Adherence to a low-risk, healthy lifestyle and risk of sudden cardiac death among women. JAMA. 2011;306:62–9.
16. Willett W, Rockström J, Loken B, Springmann M, Lang T, Vermeulen S, et al. Food in the Anthropocene: the EAT-lancet commission on healthy diets from sustainable food systems. Lancet. 2019;393:447–92.
17. Schwingshackl L, Bogensberger B, Hoffmann G. Diet quality as assessed by the Healthy Eating Index, Alternate Healthy Eating Index, Dietary Approaches to Stop Hypertension Score, and Health Outcomes: An updated systematic review and meta-analysis of cohort studies. J Acad Nutr Diet. 2018;118:74–100.e11.
18. Muszalska A, Wiecanowska J, Michałowska J, Pastusiak-Zgolińska KM, Polok I, Łompieś K, et al. The role of the planetary diet in managing metabolic syndrome and cardiovascular disease: a narrative review. Nutrients. 2025;17:862.
19. Bhandari B, Liu Z, Lin S, Macniven R, Akombi-Inyang B, Hall J, Feng X, Schutte AE, Xu X. Long-term consumption of 10 food groups and cardiovascular mortality: a systematic review and dose response meta-analysis of prospective cohort studies. Adv Nutr. 2023;14:55–63.
20. Onni AT, Balakrishna R, Perillo M, Amato M, Javadi Arjmand E, Thomassen LM, Lorenzini A, Fadnes LT. Umbrella review of systematic reviews and meta-analyses on consumption of different food groups and risk of all-cause mortality. Adv Nutr. 2025;16:100393.
21. Ganeshbabu M, Manochkumar J, Efferth T, Ramamoorthy S. Lutein: a natural defence combating age-related macular degeneration. Phytomedicine. 2025;143:156578.
22. Neyestani TR, Yari Z, Rasekhi H, Nikooyeh B. How effective are anthocyanins on healthy modification of cardiometabolic risk factors: a systematic review and meta-analysis. Diabetol Metab Syndr. 2023;15:106.
23. Sandoval-Ramírez BA, Catalán Ú, Llauradó E, Valls RM, Salamanca P, Rubió L, et al. The health benefits of anthocyanins: an umbrella review of systematic reviews and meta-analyses of observational studies and controlled clinical trials. Nutr Rev. 2022;80:1515–30.

Health Promotion and the Importance of Government Policy

9

Norman J. Temple

Abstract

- Health promotion campaigns of various types have been conducted. These are based on providing education, advice, and encouragement to the target section of the population.
- These campaigns have been carried out in communities, at worksites, and in physician offices. They have been designed to improve lifestyles in the areas of smoking, exercise, and people's diets, such as intake of fruits and vegetables. Computer-mediated health promotion through social media is now increasingly common. Major goals have been to reduce excess weight, lower the blood cholesterol, blood pressure, and blood glucose, and prevent coronary heart disease (CHD).
- Results of these campaigns have been mixed. Some have achieved very little while others have met with moderate success. Typically, target outcomes have been improved by a few percentage points and this is predicted to reduce the risk of CHD by about 5–15%.
- Government policy actions are an alternative strategy. It is likely to achieve greater success. Policies include (1) ordering a reduction in the food content of salt; (2) using taxes and subsidies to adjust the price of various foods so as to shift consumption patterns to healthier foods; and (3) policy measures to restrict advertising of unhealthy food, especially to children.
- Government policy actions are likely to meet with opposition from food corporations.

N. J. Temple (✉)
Centre for Science, Athabasca University, Athabasca, AB, Canada
e-mail: normant@athabascau.ca

N. J. Temple, T. Wilson (eds.), *Pocket Primer for Nutritional Health*,
https://doi.org/10.1007/978-3-032-25402-3_9

Introduction

It has been well established for many years that lifestyle—diet, tobacco use, exercise—has a major impact on the causation and prevention of a spectrum of diseases, namely the chronic diseases of lifestyle (CDL). The major CDL include most forms of cardiovascular disease (CVD) (including coronary heart disease (CHD), stroke, and hypertension), obesity, type 2 diabetes, and several major types of cancer. While the focus of this chapter is on nutrition in relation to health promotion and government policy, other areas are also examined especially smoking and exercise.

Health Promotion Campaigns

During the 1970s, after the intimate connection between lifestyle and health had become increasingly clear, many health professionals adopted the view that the next step was to exhort the general population to adopt a healthy lifestyle. This, hopefully, would lead to a significant improvement in population health. Here we look at various types of health promotion campaigns, most of them focused on risk factors for CVD. Most of the studies referred to here that were not computer mediated were carried out before 2012. By contrast, computer-mediated health promotion programs are much more recent.

Campaigns in Communities

Many community interventions have been carried out. There is a wide variation in the goals, the target groups, and the types of communication used in these studies. The degree of success achieved by these campaigns has been highly variable ranging from excellent success [1] to only minimal changes [2].

Worksite Health Promotion

Many interventions have been carried out at worksites. A common goal has been to improve the healthiness of the diet eaten by workers. For example, worksite canteens have displayed prominent labels to inform employees which foods are healthiest. Canteens have also increased the availability of fresh fruit and vegetables. Our best evidence is that these types of intervention can often achieve a modest improvement in the diet [3].

Health Promotion in the Physician's Office

Another setting for health promotion interventions is in medical settings such in the offices of family physicians. The targets have been diverse and have included exercise, body weight, the diet, and smoking. Overall, these interventions tended to produce modest improvements in the target measures [4].

A variation of the above trials is the targeting of patients at high risk of CHD and of other types of CDL. This is probably the most cost-effective form of intervention [5]. Two highly successful randomized controlled trials, one in the USA and one in Finland, were carried out on overweight subjects with impaired glucose tolerance, the goal being to prevent the progression to type 2 diabetes [6, 7]. The interventions consisted of physical activity and dietary change. In both studies, the estimated risk reduction was about 58%. In general, interventions focused on high-risk subjects have been more successful than other interventions [8]. This is not surprising as persons at high risk of CDL are likely to be more compliant with "doctor's orders."

Computer-Mediated Health Promotion

In recent years, many computer-mediated health promotion programs have been developed that use social media for delivering information and advice. Messages are typically delivered to the smart phones of the target people. This is a diverse field with programs focused on exercise, diet, obesity, and smoking. Promising findings have been reported from many interventions [9–11].

Health Promotion and the Individual

What the above projects demonstrate is that appealing to individuals to change their lifestyles achieves only limited success. This might be expected to reduce the risk of CVD (including CHD) by about 5–15%. While this is certainly beneficial, it will not affect the majority of people at risk. We can confidently predict, therefore, that exhortations to the individual, whether via the community (including in schools), at the worksite, in the physician's office, or via the mass media or social media, will not achieve a major impact on the numbers of people succumbing to CDL.

Unfortunately, it is not clear which strategies are most likely to lead to at least moderate success. Findings suggest that success is more likely with interventions that target adults rather than children and with those that use multiple types of information and encouragement interventions rather than a single type [12].

Is the Population Adopting a Healthier Lifestyle?

The limited effectiveness of health promotion is confirmed by another line of evidence. From the 1970s onward, enormous amounts of dietary information and advice have been disseminated to the populations of all Western countries. People have been exposed to many thousands of TV programs, articles in newspapers and magazines, and books. Governments have made dietary information, such as food guides, widely available. Food packages now carry labels that provide nutrition information on the food. Yet, despite all this effort, relatively little progress has been made in persuading the general population to follow the recommended dietary changes. This is demonstrated by the findings from surveys of the American diet as indicated by the following surveys.

- Almost 60% of calorie intake in the USA comes from ultra-processed foods [13]. This is also the case in the UK [14]. As explained in Chap. 4, most of these foods are unhealthy.
- A detailed analysis of diets eaten in the USA reported some improvement in the diets eaten by American adults between 1999 and 2020. Nevertheless, 37.4% of adults were consuming a "poor" diet. This was defined as less than 40% adherence to the recommended diet. Fewer than 1 in 50 were consuming an "ideal" diet, defined as at least an 80% adherence to dietary recommendations [15].

An overview of the above evidence compels the conclusion that the majority of Americans largely ignore advice to lead a healthy lifestyle, especially with regard to their diet.

Why Are People Resistant to Education, Advice, and Encouragement?

"Education, advice, and encouragement" is a convenient term that covers diverse approaches, including health promotion, that aim to persuade people to adopt a healthier lifestyle [16].

Most readers of this chapter probably have a mindset that health is of great importance and that everyone should therefore try their best to follow a healthy lifestyle. But, clearly, the majority of the population give their health a much lower priority. How can we explain this?

Myriad factors influence people's behavior besides concerns about how to protect health. Social factors, such as housing, employment, and income, shape people's attitudes as does their education. Advertising directly affects what people want while prices and income determine whether they can afford it. We are also creatures of habit and custom; resistance may therefore be expected when lifestyle modification requires changes in longstanding behavior and goes against fashion or peer pressure. We must also bear in mind that individuals have little control over many aspects of their physical environment, such as pollution, food contamination, and where and what kinds of foods are sold and the cost of it. It is probably naïve, therefore, to expect dramatic results from interventions that merely exhort the individual to lead a healthier lifestyle. In other words, a strategy that aims to improve population health by using education, advice, and encouragement is likely to be of modest value but is very unlikely to lead to a major improvement in population health.

This frustrating problem can be stated as follows: you can lead a horse to water, but you can't make it wear a swimsuit.

Government Policy

A strategy that has a serious chance of success must start with the recognition that it is the environment around us that plays a major role in determining the lifestyles of the general population. The word "environment" here refers to the many factors that affect our behavior and our diet. Factors of major importance in the area of diet include food composition, food prices, and food marketing. From this it follows that in order to achieve a substantial reduction in the scourge of chronic diseases of lifestyle, it is essential that policies are implemented so as to change the environment. In other words, we need to radically change the environment from one that encourages people to follow an unhealthy lifestyle to one that fosters a healthy lifestyle. This requires important changes in a range of government policies, regulations, and laws. These policies are referred to here as "action policies."

The Case for Action Policies

Attention is now turned to a strategy designed to improve the nutrition quality of the diets consumed by the population, namely action policies carried out by direct action by governments. There are sound reasons to believe that this strategy can be a very effective tool for improving the national diet and population health. These arguments were presented in a recent paper [16]. Another recent paper presented proposals for how this strategy could be adapted to the specific problem of the obesity epidemic [17].

Action policies by governments in the area of public health have a long history. Many such policies were implemented in the nineteenth century and achieved great success. Deadly infectious diseases, including cholera and typhoid, were brought under control by such measures as providing the population with safe drinking water as well as sewage disposal. This approach continued in the twentieth century with many new policies. For example, in recent decades, it became compulsory for cars to be fitted with seat belts and for these to be used by anyone riding in a car. Smoking in many public places has been banned. This prevents the harm caused by second-hand smoke.

Until the 1970s, hazardous amounts of lead were present in various consumer products, including gasoline and paint. Governments in many countries, including the USA, forced major reductions or removal of lead from these products. In the case of lead in gasoline, there was strong opposition from the petroleum industry. Fortunately, governments resisted this pressure. These measures greatly reduced the amount of lead that entered the environment including the air. Testing of American children revealed that their blood concentration of lead fell by at least 75% between the late 1970s and the early1990s [18, 19].

Action Policies in the Area of Nutrition

This strategy has been applied to the field of nutrition. Many regulations have been implemented over the decades in the area of food safety. Likewise, it became compulsory for particular micronutrients to be added to some foods, such as the addition of vitamin D to milk and of thiamin to bread. In 1996, the USA and Canada implemented a policy that mandated the addition of folic acid to grain products. The goal was to correct low intake of the vitamin in pregnant women and thereby prevent spina bifida in infants. This policy and the others mentioned above have generally achieved a high degree of success. Moreover, the policies, in most cases, are highly cost-effective.

Removal of *Trans*-Fatty Acids from Food

Around the years 2010 to 2018, the USA and Canada implemented a policy that forced food manufacturers to remove *trans*-fatty acids from food. Other countries implemented similar policies but with more modest targets [20]. The rationale for this policy was the discovery that consumption of these fats significantly increases the risk of CHD [21]. These unnatural fats are formed during the production of hydrogenated fats. Until their removal, major foods sources included hard margarine, cakes, doughnuts, cookies, and deep-fried foods.

Reducing the Salt Content of Food

Salt is another substance in food where a strong case can be made for an action policy so as to reduce intake. The populations of the USA and most other Western countries consume about 50% to 100% more than the recommended amount [22]. As detailed in Chap. 3, this excessive intake increases the risk of hypertension and cardiovascular disease. This indicates that a reduction of one-third in the salt content of food could help prevent many thousands of cases of CVD.

The only practical way to achieve that goal is to greatly reduce the salt content of processed food as that is the source of roughly 75–80% of dietary salt [23]. One strategy is voluntary action by industry [24], a policy adopted by the UK [25]. In the nine years following the implementation of the campaign (2008 to 2017), salt intake by adults in the UK fell by about 16% [26]. This is far less than the required one-third reduction. An action policy approach similar to that adopted to reduce the food content of *trans*-fatty acids (i.e., setting mandatory limits on the salt content of processed food) could achieve the required reduction in salt intake in a mere few years.

Action Policies in Schools

Schools are fertile ground for action policies. For example, vast numbers of American schools have vending machines that sell unhealthy foods or beverages. Evidence reveals that when action is taken to improve the food environment in schools, such as by ensuring that vending machines stock only healthy foods and that meals served in schools are of high nutritional quality, students then consume a healthier diet [27]. Some jurisdictions in the USA and in other countries have implemented concrete policies in order to achieve these goals. For example, in 2011, Spain banned unhealthy food from schools [28].

A study that is worthy of attention is Romp and Chomp [29]. This was a community-wide, multisetting, multistrategy intervention conducted on 12,000 young children in Australia from 2004 to 2008. The goals were to reduce the prevalence of obesity by improving diets and encouraging children to engage in more exercise. The intervention achieved much success.

Taxes and Subsidies as Tools to Change Food Prices

It is well known that when the price of a product is increased, sales go down, and vice versa. Economists refer to this phenomenon as price elasticity. Many studies have demonstrated that this rule applies to tobacco and alcohol. It also applies to food. For example, when fruit in a supermarket is starting to become overripe, the store will lower the price in order to sell the produce quickly.

This rule can be put to good use in order to achieve an impact on the national diet [30, 31]. This means manipulating food prices as follows:

1. A tax can be added to less healthy choices, such as white bread and sugar-sweetened beverages (SSB), so as to increase the price.
2. Subsidies can be applied to healthy foods, such as fruit, vegetables, and wholegrain cereals, in order to lower the price.

As a rule, an increase in the price of unhealthy foods of 10% will lower intake by 6%, while a price reduction of 10% on healthy foods will increase consumption by 12% [32]. If the level of subsidies and taxes are carefully regulated, then the cost to the government should be minimal as money spent on subsidies will be canceled out by the extra revenue from taxes. Similarly, there should be no overall effect on food prices.

It is in relation to SSB where this strategy has attracted most attention. Indeed, several cities in the USA and about 90 countries have implemented a tax on SSB [33].

Food Prices and Socioeconomic Status

The question of food prices is especially important in relation to people who have a low socioeconomic status. Many studies have demonstrated that people on a low income have the least healthy diets. They also tend to have the poorest health and the highest prevalence of obesity. This is a complex issue with multiple factors at work. But one important factor that pressures poorer people to eat a less healthy diet than do more affluent people is that healthier diets are generally more expensive than unhealthy diets [34]. For example, obtaining calories from fruits and vegetables is much more costly than buying calories from foods rich in added sugar [35]. Likewise, a study in Belgium concluded that buying food energy in the form of unprocessed or minimally processed foods costs more than twice as much as buying it from ultraprocessed food (1.29 vs 0.55 euros per 100 kcal) [36].

These findings lend extra weight to the argument that making healthy foods more affordable will improve the national diet and thereby improve population health.

Another strategy that can help poorer people to obtain healthy foods is to distribute vouchers that can be exchanged for healthy foods. These are often referred to as "food stamps" in the USA.

Food Advertising

Children are on the receiving end of an enormous amount of food advertising. Traditionally, this has come mostly via TV but an increasing share now comes by way of social media. The vast majority is for unhealthy foods or for fast-food restaurants. Such advertising is often successful in inducing children to consume the advertised foods [37]. In particular, these adverts induce children to consume more snacks, sweetened beverages, and fast food [38, 39]. Moreover, exposure to such advertising is associated with the risk of poorer health and obesity in children and adolescents [39, 40].

The case is therefore strong for a ban on advertising for unhealthy foods where children are a major target. In order to make this policy effective in the area of TV, the ban would have to cover all programs being shown late into the evening as a great many children are still watching TV at that hour. As far as it is practical, this policy needs to be extended to other forms of marketing. There is evidence that such bans can be effective. According to one analysis, a ban on TV advertising in the USA would lead to a roughly 19% decrease in the numbers of children and adolescents eating two or more fast food meals per week and would lead to a modest decrease in obesity rates [41]. Many jurisdictions in different countries have banned adverts that encourage young people to eat unhealthy food [33].

Other Action Policies

Research studies indicate that several other action policies show potential for helping to improve the population diet. These include policies that aim to reduce the availability of unhealthy food in food establishments (as well as in schools) and policies that mandate changes to portion sizes and the size of food packages [32].

The Question of Cost-Effectiveness

Despite being limited in its impact, health promotion that relies on education, advice, and encouragement, is, nevertheless, of much value. This extends to considerations of cost. Because minor changes in the lifestyle of millions of people can make valuable contributions to public health, expenditure on health promotion can be cost-effective [42, 43]. The evidence is especially strong with health promotion at the worksite. This was demonstrated by a review carried out by the American Heart Association. As interventions at the worksite can bring about a reduction in absenteeism and improved productivity, nutrition programs can be highly cost-effective, saving employers several dollars for each dollar invested [44].

Compared with health promotion it can be confidently asserted that action policies carried out by the government can have an even larger impact at relatively modest cost. As a result they can be highly cost-effective. This was clearly demonstrated with analyses of the cost and health benefits of policies that reduce the food content of *trans*-fatty acids and salt [45, 46].

The Problem of Food Corporations

The food industry profits enormously from the sale of highly processed food. For that reason, food corporations and their lobbyists endeavor to construct barriers to the implementation of effective policies of the type proposed here [47]. These corporations are emulating the game plan developed decades ago by the tobacco industry. The pressure exerted by the food industry in protection of its financial welfare is explored in Chap. 14.

Conclusions

This chapter has briefly analyzed two strategies for combating the chronic diseases of lifestyle and enhancing population health. Table 9.1 summarizes these strategies.

One strategy, health promotion, employs education, advice, and encouragement. This strategy has met with only limited success. Nevertheless, this strategy is still of much value. The alternative strategy is based on developing and implementing government policies, regulations, and laws with the goal of changing the current environment in areas that affect health. With respect to diet, the current environment encourages people to consume an unhealthy diet. Instead, policies need to be implemented that change the food environment so that the population consumes a healthier diet. These "action policies" may include mandating a reduction in the salt content of food, using taxes and subsidies so as to encourage the purchase and consumption of healthier food, and restricting the advertising of unhealthy food, especially to children.

Section 6 of Chap. 15 takes the above strategies for improving population health one step further. These strategies are combined into a single plan referred to as a "strategic plan." This comprehensive action plan has the potential to achieve a major advance in population health.

Table 9.1 Summary of key features of health promotion and action policies by governments

Health promotion campaigns based on education, advice, and encouragement	
Target groups	Whole community (including schools)
	Employees at worksites
	Patients in physicians' offices
	Persons using social media (especially smart phones)
Tactics used	Communication via mass media
	Face-to-face communication
	Delivering information and advice via social media (especially smart phones)
Goals	Improve diet
	More exercise
	Lose weight
	Quit smoking
Degree of success	Varies between very low and moderate (expected to reduce risk of CVD by 5–15%)
Government policy actions (policies, regulations, laws)	
Goal	Change food environment in order to change population behavior toward a healthier diet
Examples	Order a reduction in food content of salt
	Increase availability of healthy food, restrict availability of unhealthy food
	Use taxes and subsidies so that a healthy diet is more affordable than an unhealthy diet
	Ban advertisements for unhealthy food especially to children
Expected degree of success	High
Other potential advantage(s)	Likely to be highly cost-effective
Potential disadvantage(s)	Opposition from food corporations

References

1. Vartiainen E, Laatikainen T, Peltonen M, Juolevi A, Männistö S, Sundvall J, et al. Thirty-five-year trends in cardiovascular risk factors in Finland. Int J Epidemiol. 2010;39:504–18.
2. Winkleby MA, Feldman HA, Murray DM. Joint analysis of three U.S. community intervention trials for reduction of cardiovascular risk. J Clin Epidemiol. 1997;50:645–58.
3. Virtanen M, Lallukka T, Elovainio M, Steptoe A, Kivimäki M. Effectiveness of workplace interventions for health promotion. Lancet Public Health. 2025;10:e512–30.
4. Wilcox S, Parra-Medina D, Thompson-Robinson M, Will J. Nutrition and physical activity interventions to reduce cardiovascular disease risk in health care settings: a quantitative review with a focus on women. Nutr Rev. 2001;59:197–214.
5. Field K, Thorogood M, Silagy C, Normand C, O'Neill C, Muir J. Strategies for reducing coronary risk factors in primary care: which is most cost effective? BMJ. 1995;310:1109–12.
6. Tuomilehto J, Lindstrom J, Eriksson JG, Valle TT, Hämäläinen H, Ilanne-Parikka P, et al. Prevention of type 2 diabetes mellitus by changes in lifestyle among subjects with impaired glucose tolerance. N Engl J Med. 2001;344:1343–50.

7. Knowler WC, Barrett-Connor E, Fowler SE, Hamman RF, Lachin JM, Walker EA, et al. Reduction in the incidence of type 2 diabetes with lifestyle intervention or metformin. N Engl J Med. 2002;346:393–403.
8. Ammerman AS, Lindquist CH, Lohr KN, Hersey J. The efficacy of behavioral interventions to modify dietary fat and fruit and vegetable intake: a review of the evidence. Prev Med. 2002;35:25–41.
9. Stellefson M, Paige SR, Chaney BH, Chaney JD. Evolving role of social media in health promotion: updated responsibilities for health education specialists. Int J Environ Res Public Health. 2020;17:1153.
10. Patel RM, Cohen N, De Lucca M, Serna CA. Leveraging social media for population health promotion: evaluation of a year-long nonprofit public health campaign. Cureus. 2026;18:e105854.
11. Vanwinkelen K, Spruyt B, Smits T. Digital interventions targeting healthy and sustainable eating behavior: systematic review and meta-analysis. J Med Internet Res. 2026;28:e80821.
12. Kachwaha S, Kim SS, Das JK, Rasheed S, Gavaravarapu SM, Pandey RP. Behavior change interventions to address unhealthy food consumption: a scoping review. Curr Dev Nutr. 2024;8:102104.
13. Juul F, Parekh N, Martinez-Steele E, Monteiro CA, Chang VW. Ultra-processed food consumption among US adults from 2001 to 2018. Am J Clin Nutr. 2022;115:211–21.
14. Rauber F, da Costa Louzada ML, Steele EM, Millett C, Monteiro CA, Levy RB. Ultra-processed food consumption and chronic non-communicable diseases-related dietary nutrient profile in the UK (2008-2014). Nutrients. 2018;10:pii E587.
15. Liu J, Mozaffarian D. Trends in diet quality among U.S. adults from 1999 to 2020 by race, ethnicity, and socioeconomic disadvantage. Ann Intern Med. 2024;177:841–50.
16. Temple NJ. A comparison of strategies to improve population diets: government policy versus education and advice. J Nutr Metab. 2020;2020:5932516.
17. Temple NJ. A proposed strategy against obesity: how government policy can counter the obesogenic environment. Nutrients. 2023;15:2910.
18. Pirkle JL, Brody DJ, Gunter EW, Kramer RA, Paschal DC, Flegal KM, et al. The decline in blood lead levels in the United States. JAMA. 1994;272:284–91.
19. Brody DJ, Pirkle JL, Kramer RA, Flegal KM, Matte TD, Gunter EW, et al. Blood lead levels in the US population. JAMA. 1994;272:277–83.
20. Ghebreyesus TA, Frieden TR. REPLACE: a roadmap to make the world trans fat free by 2023. Lancet. 2018;391:1978–80.
21. de Souza RJ, Mente A, Maroleanu A, Cozma AJ, Ha V, Kishibe T, et al. Intake of saturated and trans unsaturated fatty acids and risk of all cause mortality, cardiovascular disease, and type 2 diabetes: systematic review and meta-analysis of observational studies. BMJ. 2015;351:h3978.
22. Drewnowski A, Rehm CD, Maillot M, Mendoza A, Monsivais P. The feasibility of meeting the WHO guidelines for sodium and potassium: a cross-national comparison study. BMJ Open. 2015;5:e006625.
23. Hooper L, Bartlett C, Davey SG, Ebrahim S. Advice to reduce dietary salt for prevention of cardiovascular disease. Cochrane Database Syst Rev. 2004:CD003656.
24. Rosewarne E, Santos JA, Trieu K, Tekle D, Mhurchu CN, Jones A, et al. A global review of national strategies to reduce sodium concentrations in packaged foods. Adv Nutr. 2022;13:1820–33.
25. Temple NJ. Population strategies to reduce sodium intake: the right way and the wrong way. Nutrition. 2011;27:387.
26. Gressier M, Sassi F, Frost G. Contribution of reformulation, product renewal, and changes in consumer behavior to the reduction of salt intakes in the UK population between 2008/2009 and 2016/2017. Am J Clin Nutr. 2021;114:1092–9.
27. Micha R, Karageorgou D, Bakogianni I, Trichia E, Whitsel LP, Story M, et al. Effectiveness of school food environment policies on children's dietary behaviors: A systematic review and meta-analysis. PLoS One. 2018;13:e0194555.

28. deLago M. Spain bans sale of unhealthy food in schools in bid to tackle obesity. BMJ. 2011;342:d4073.
29. de Silva-Sanigorski AM, Bell AC, Kremer P, Nichols M, Crellin M, Smith M, et al. Reducing obesity in early childhood: results from Romp & Chomp, an Australian community-wide intervention program. Am J Clin Nutr. 2010;91:831–40.
30. Gittelsohn J, Trude ACB, Kim H. Pricing strategies to encourage availability, purchase, and consumption of healthy foods and beverages: a systematic review. Prev Chronic Dis. 2017;14:E107.
31. Valizadeh P, Ng SW. Promoting healthier purchases: ultraprocessed food taxes and minimally processed foods subsidies for the low income. Am J Prev Med. 2024;67:3–14.
32. Hansen KL, Golubovic S, Eriksen CU, Jørgensen T, Toft U. Effectiveness of food environment policies in improving population diets: a review of systematic reviews. Eur J Clin Nutr. 2022;76:637–46.
33. Forray AI, Borzan CM. Implementation of national nutrition policies and strategies to reduce unhealthy diets: an ecological analysis of 194 countries from 2017 to 2021. Nutrients. 2024;16:911.
34. Pedroni C, Castetbon K, Desbouys L, Rouche M, Vandevijvere S. The cost of diets according to nutritional quality and sociodemographic characteristics: a population-based assessment in Belgium. J Acad Nutr Diet. 2021;121:2187–200.e4.
35. Drewnowski A. Obesity and the food environment: dietary energy density and diet costs. Am J Prev Med. 2004;27(3 Suppl):154–62.
36. Vandevijvere S, Pedroni C, De Ridder K, Castetbon K. The cost of diets according to their caloric share of ultraprocessed and minimally processed foods in Belgium. Nutrients. 2020;12:2787.
37. Wiecha JL, Peterson KE, Ludwig DS, Kim J, Sobol A, Gortmaker SL. When children eat what they watch: impact of television viewing on dietary intake in youth. Arch Pediatr Adolesc Med. 2006;160:436.
38. Smith R, Kelly B, Yeatman H, Boyland E. Food marketing influences children's attitudes, preferences and consumption: a systematic critical review. Nutrients. 2019;11:875.
39. Zimmerman FJ, Bell JF. Association of television content type and obesity in children. Am J Public Health. 2010;100:334–40.
40. Harris JL, Taillie LS. More than a nuisance: implications of food marketing for public health efforts to curb childhood obesity. Annu Rev Public Health. 2024;45:213–33.
41. Kristensen AH, Flottemesch TJ, Maciosek MV, Jenson J, Barclay G, Ashe M, et al. Reducing childhood obesity through U.S. federal policy: a microsimulation analysis. Am J Prev Med. 2014;47:604–12.
42. Aldana SG. Financial impact of health promotion programs: a comprehensive review of the literature. Am J Health Promot. 2001;15:296–320.
43. Golaszewski T. Shining lights: studies that have most influenced the understanding of health promotion's financial impact. Am J Health Promot. 2001;15:332–40.
44. Carnethon M, Whitsel LP, Franklin BA, Kris-Etherton P, Milani R, Pratt CA, et al. Worksite wellness programs for cardiovascular disease prevention: a policy statement from the American Heart Association. Circulation. 2009;120:1725–41.
45. Marklund M, Zheng M, Veerman JL, Wu JHY. Estimated health benefits, costs, and cost-effectiveness of eliminating industrial trans-fatty acids in Australia: A modelling study. PLoS Med. 2020;17:e1003407.
46. Palar K, Sturm R. Potential societal savings from reduced sodium consumption in the U.S. adult population. Am J Health Promot. 2009;24:49–57.
47. Gilmore AB, Fabbri A, Baum F, Bertscher A, Bondy K, Chang HJ, et al. Defining and conceptualising the commercial determinants of health. Lancet. 2023;401:1194–213.

Front-of-Package Food Labels: Their Types, History, Impact on Consumer Behavior, and Support by Digital Technologies

10

Nikola Ljusic

Abstract

- Front-of-package food labels transform nutritional data into simplified logos or symbols and are placed on products to help consumers choose healthier options.
- They can be classified as reductive nutrient-specific or interpretative labels. They may present graded, single, or percentage-based evaluations of the healthfulness
- Initially, most of these labels were single summary labels and voluntary. Currently, there exist more mandatory labels, graded summary labels in Europe, and warning labels in the Americas.
- Most labels impact consumer behavior positively, and graded summary labels seem promising. However, their impact is relatively small in real purchase situations and on the quality of the diet
- Digital technologies may support FOP labeling by labeling products in novel ways.

This chapter is based on research from the author's doctoral project at the Kristiania University of Applied Sciences, School of Economics, Innovation, and Technology, Behavior and Technology Lab.

N. Ljusic (✉)
Behavior and Technology Lab, Kristiania University of Applied Sciences, Oslo, Norway
e-mail: nikola@ljusic.com; Nikola.Ljusic@kristiania.no

N. J. Temple, T. Wilson (eds.), *Pocket Primer for Nutritional Health*,
https://doi.org/10.1007/978-3-032-25402-3_10

Introduction

Unhealthy food consumption is a major problem affecting countries worldwide, companies, and consumers. For countries, unhealthy foods are costly due to their impact on obesity and many other diseases. They especially affect vulnerable populations. For instance, an unbalanced diet is a significant cause of obesity and overweight [1]; half of adults and one in three children are overweight [2]. The global economic burden of obesity is estimated at about US$3 trillion per year [1]. There is a link between diet and mental health [3].

The food industry now faces increased pressure from various organizations and countries proposing strict approaches, including bans, taxation, and marketing restrictions on unhealthy foods [4]. Many countries have adopted nutritional policies to combat diet-related non-communicable diseases, though not without challenges [5]. Companies may lose revenue when consumers' needs and wants are not met. Several studies indicate that consumers are willing to pay a premium price for healthier food products [6]. Hence, there are some incentives for companies to promote healthier foods.

It is crucial that knowledge from nutritional science should be applied to promote healthy food choices among consumers in a pragmatic manner, including at the point of purchase. Several strategies have been proposed, each with unique benefits and challenges.

Front-of-package (FOP) food labels are one proposed strategy that has several benefits. FOP labels are symbols or logos placed on products to indicate to consumers the healthiness of the products, either as an overall summary or according to their specific nutrients [7, 8]. They differ from back-of-package nutritional declarations (e.g., Fig. 10.1) by presenting simplified nutritional information on the front of the package (e.g., Fig. 10.2). Numerous countries have developed or implemented FOP labeling systems, and there are now many such labeling systems [11–14]. There are several benefits of such labels, including: the potential to increase healthy food choices while not restricting product options; implementing them may be cost-effective; and they could transform nutritional data into simplified information through logos or labels that reduce evaluation efforts for consumers. However, several challenges remain, including the use of different labels in different countries, the fact that many consumers are not familiar with these labels and which products have these labels, and they do not automatically lead to an increase in the purchase or consumption of healthier foods [15]. Specifically, their effectiveness may depend on several factors, including the type of behavior being measured, the type of labeling used, other product-related factors, and the situational factors being investigated. It is crucial to investigate how these labels can reliably influence consumers' behavior as the effectiveness of these labels depends on whether consumers use them.

This chapter provides a brief overview of FOP food labeling. First, it will describe several types of FOP labeling systems. Second, the historical development of these labels across countries will be described. Third, the impact of these labels and other factors on consumer behavior will be examined. Lastly, how these labels may be supported by using digital technologies will also be discussed.

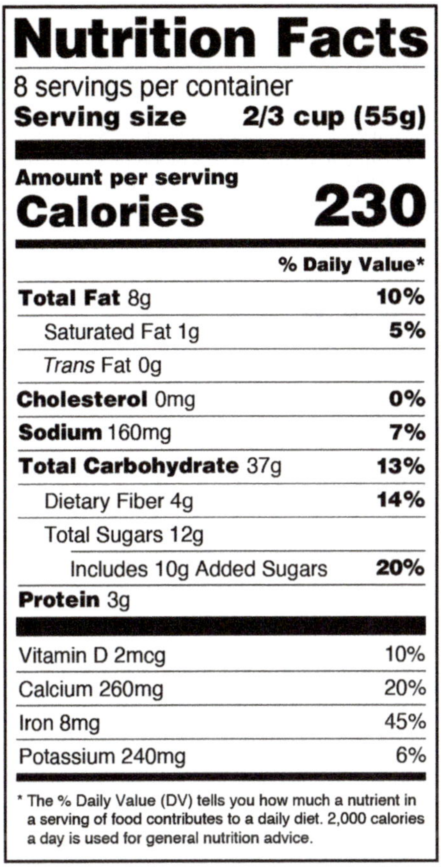
Nutrition Facts
8 servings per container
Serving size 2/3 cup (55g)
Amount per serving
Calories 230
% Daily Value*
Total Fat 8g 10%
Saturated Fat 1g 5%
Trans Fat 0g
Cholesterol 0mg 0%
Sodium 160mg 7%
Total Carbohydrate 37g 13%
Dietary Fiber 4g 14%
Total Sugars 12g
Includes 10g Added Sugars 20%
Protein 3g
Vitamin D 2mcg 10%
Calcium 260mg 20%
Iron 8mg 45%
Potassium 240mg 6%
* The % Daily Value (DV) tells you how much a nutrient in a serving of food contributes to a daily diet. 2,000 calories a day is used for general nutrition advice.

Fig. 10.1 Nutrition Facts label. The Nutrition Facts label is found on the back or the side of food packages. (Source: U.S. Food and Drug Administration [9])

Fig. 10.2 Nordic Keyhole label. The Nordic Keyhole is a type of single summary label. (Source: Swedish Food Agency [10])

The Diverse Types of Front-of-Package Food Labels

There exist many FOP food labels [e.g., 16, 17]. They have six common characteristics, namely: (a) graphical labels placed on the front of the package; (b) transform nutritional data to simplified information using symbols or logos; (c) present an overall summary, nutrient-specific information, or combined information; (d) can be used across different products; (e) present this information on products based on different labeling rules and requirements; and (f) aim to help consumers to identify healthier food choices. The essential feature of labels is that they focus on the entire product or its nutrients using standardized criteria with the goal of helping consumers to assess products by reducing the time and effort required to find and transform nutritional data into simplified information.

The types of FOP food labels can be classified into reductive and interpretative labels [8, 11, 18], and further into summary, nutrient-specific, or combined labels [7, 19], providing graded, single, or percentage-based information regarding the nutritional value of products (Fig. 10.3). Reductive labels display key nutrients on the front of the package in a descriptive manner without explicitly suggesting the healthfulness of each nutrient. Interpretive labels display information about whether the product is healthy, either according to an overall summary indicator of the product or its nutrient-specific content. Summary indicators may incorporate an overall assessment of nutrients in their algorithm. Graded labels present a score ranging from a maximum to a minimum value, while single labels are binary, indicating the healthiness of a product by its presence or absence. Percentage-based labels indicate the degree of healthiness of a product in percentage terms relative to a reference category and are often nutrient-specific.

There are several examples of these types of FOP labels. Examples of graded summary labels (i.e., rating labels) are the Nutri-Score and Guiding Stars. The Nutri-Score label assigns one of five grades, from the healthiest (A) to the unhealthiest (E), accompanied by green, yellow, and red colors in that order (Fig. 10.4). The

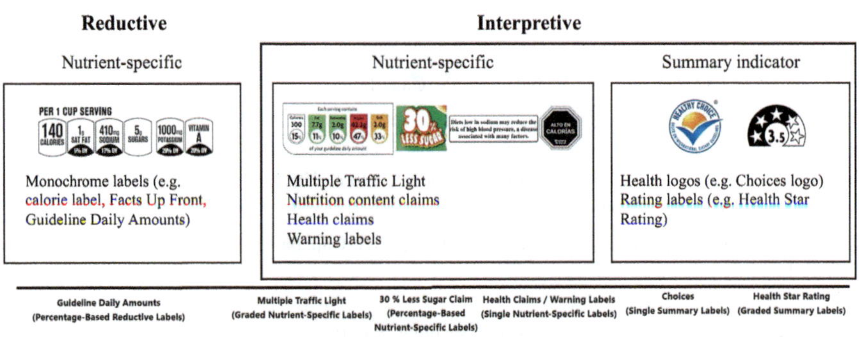

Fig. 10.3 Examples of FOP labels. (Adapted from Ikonen et al. [8] with modifications. The image on the left is a Guideline Daily Amounts label. The central image depicts a Multiple Traffic Lights label on the left and a warning label on the right. The image on the right depicts the Choices label on the left and a Health Star Rating label on the right)

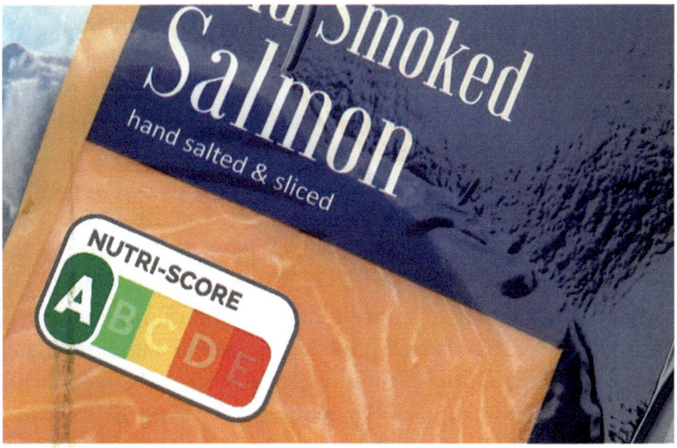

Fig. 10.4 Nutri-Score label. The Nutri-Score is a type of graded summary label. (Source: Istockphoto.com/Cebas [20])

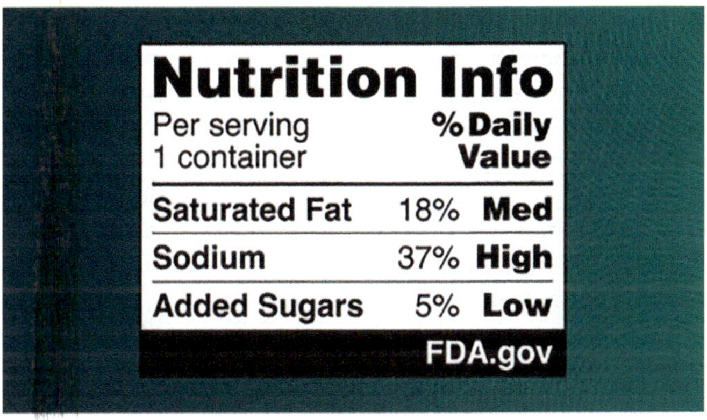

Fig. 10.5 The U.S. Food and Drug Administration's Proposed Label. The U.S. Food and Drug Administration's Proposed Label is a type of percentage-based reductive label. (Source: U.S. Food and Drug Administration [21])

Guiding Stars label does this by presenting stars ranging from three to no stars. Examples of single summary labels (i.e., health logos) include the Nordic Keyhole (Fig. 10.2), the Choices label (Fig. 10.3), the Finnish Heart Symbol, and the Heart Foundation Tick, among others, which are often placed on the healthiest products within their respective food categories, although with varying requirements.

Many nutrient-specific labels exist, both reductive and interpretive. Examples of reductive labels are Guideline Daily Amounts (Fig. 10.3), NutrInform Battery, Facts Up Front, Reference Intake, and calorie labels. Examples of graded nutrient-specific labels include the Multiple Traffic Lights (Fig. 10.3) and the proposed U.S. label (Fig. 10.5). These display key nutrients on the front of products and state if the content is high, medium, or low. As with Multiple Traffic Lights, the value for each nutrient is colored red (high, least healthy), yellow (medium), or green (low, most healthy).

Warning labels are a type of interpretive single nutrient-specific label. They include words such as "High in Salt" and "High in Sugar" (Fig. 10.3). This design has been adopted in several such countries. Many food packages have a nutritional content claim such as "High in Fiber" or "No Added Sugar". Like warning labels they are a single nutrient-specific label, but they have the opposite goal, namely to encourage purchase rather than to discourage it. Percentage-based labels include logos such as "30% Less Sugar". Lastly, an example of a combined label is the Health Star Rating (Fig. 10.3) which provides an overall summary indicator of the entire product, ranging from the healthiest (five stars) to the least healthy (half a star), and also displays evaluations of key nutrients in terms of "Low" to "High".

The diverse types of FOP food labels differ in their strengths and weaknesses. Summary labels offer a single evaluation [22]. This has the advantage of being easier for consumers to understand and requires less knowledge. Graded labels provide more nuanced evaluations than single labels. With single labels, consumers may mistakenly believe that labeled products are significantly healthier than unlabeled products when, in reality, the differences between two products may be minor.

Nutrient-specific labels shift the focus from the entire product to a few key nutrients. This increases the effort needed by consumers to evaluate the information presented and this may cause some confusion [22]. This may be problematic for fats and saturated fats. Nutrient-specific labels often include these nutrients, and many consumers avoid them due to health concerns. However, various fat-rich foods, such as olive oil, nuts, and fish, are protective against various diseases. Likewise, the intake of saturated fats is of much less importance in the causation of heart disease than was previously believed [23].

Let us review the strengths and weaknesses of these FOP labels. The most used graded summary label is Nutri-Score, which considers many ingredients in the food, such as fruit, vegetables, fiber, and other components. The overall summary (i.e., letters from A to E) is therefore based on the overall healthiness of the food. Nutrient-specific labels include the Multiple Traffic Lights and Guideline Daily Amounts. These focus on a few nutrients rather than the food as a whole. As a result, consumers may be misled regarding whether the food is healthy. This may be the case when nutrients such as fat and saturated fat are included. Hence, Nutri-Score is likely to be a better indicator of the overall healthiness of a food than nutrient-specific labels.

History of Implementation of Front-of-Package Food Labels

Attention is now turned to the history of the implementation of FOP food labels across countries. The overall trends indicate that the majority of FOP labeling initially consisted of positive single summary labels, followed by more implementation of nutrient-specific labels, and then warning labels and graded summary labels

[13]. Initially, most of these labels were voluntary, but mandatory labeling is now increasing [12–14].

The first modern FOP label was the Heart Guide Symbol from the United States, which was introduced in 1987 and later revised as the Heart-Check Certification in 1995. Its usage of the heart symbol later became common in other labeling designs. The Nordic Keyhole was one of the earliest FOP labels to be adopted in several countries. Sweden initially implemented it in 1989, but other Nordic countries later adopted it, followed by some non-Nordic countries. The Heart Foundational Tick was first introduced in Australia, followed by New Zealand, but was discontinued in 2016, partially due to the later introduction of another label. After 1989, several country-specific FOP labels emerged. Slovenia implemented a Heart Foundation Symbol, "Za Srce", meaning "For the Heart". South Africa implemented its Heart Mark Logo. The Canadian Health Check instead had a tick that was implemented in 1999 but withdrawn in 2014. The Finnish Heart Symbol was introduced in 2000. Following that, the Choices label was implemented in several Central European countries and also had a tick.

The exceptions to the single summary labels were the mandatory warning label "High Salt" in Finland. The Multiple Traffic Lights system was added to food packages in the United Kingdom in 2004. It was then adopted in several other European Union countries. Graded summary labels such as the Guiding Stars and NuVal from the United States were implemented later [24].

There have been many developments with FOP labels in recent years. Reductive labels such as Reference Intakes and Facts Up Front (Fig. 10.3) were introduced in the European Union and the United States. The Guideline Daily Amounts was adopted in Mexico but was revised in 2015. The "High in" warning label with a black octagon was launched in Chile in 2016 and then in other countries in the Americas. Different designs of the warning label were introduced, such as a magnifying glass in Brazil and Canada.

More recently, Nutri-Score appeared in France in 2017, followed by Belgium, Switzerland, Portugal, Germany, Spain, and the Netherlands. Single summary labels were implemented in China and other countries in 2019. Additionally, the Guiding Stars design was revised in the United States in 2021. The combined label Health Star Rating was introduced by Australia and New Zealand in 2014.

Consumer Behavior and Front-of-Package Food Labels

FOP food labels are intended to help consumers choose healthier products. Most studies indicate that FOP labels have a positive impact on consumers' behavior, although this effect is much diminished in real-world purchasing situations [15]. There are many variables involved, including aspects related to the label, other product-related factors, and consumer characteristics (e.g., gender, age, and socioeconomic status) [13].

Consumer behavior is broad [25], and several behaviors have been investigated concerning FOP food labels. These include purchases, consumption, attention, and subjective measures [8, 15, 19, 26–28]. The purchase of total products, healthy products, unhealthy products, products by food category, and labeled products has been researched. These are recorded by using retailer software, receipts, observational data, and video cameras [15]. Defining healthy foods may be based on nutrient content and ratings by experts [15]. However, the majority of studies have measured the impact of FOP labels by asking subjects which food they would choose to buy when shown images of different foods or of actual foods in a laboratory setting [29]. Attention—whether consumers are drawn to certain stimuli [19]—can be measured in terms of the presentation of some tasks involving multiple stimuli and consumers' reaction time. Presenting products with different labeling systems but the same nutritional information, such as reductive vs. interpretative nutrient-specific labels, could lead to different fixation times or accuracy when answering questions about the product [13] or affect the viewing of Nutrition Facts labels [8]. Various subjective measures are also studied. These include evaluations made by participants without necessarily wishing to buy or consume particular products, along with reported perceptions of healthiness, tastiness, health risks, and product attitudes [19, 30]. For example, identifying healthy products can be measured by ranking the nutritional quality of foods, quiz scores, ratings on a 10-point scale, the percentage of correct responses for the healthiest food option among several possible responses, and identifying the least healthy product [7].

There are many studies on consumer behavior concerning FOP labels, other product-related factors [13], and situational factors. The presence of FOP labels generally has a positive impact on purchase, attention, and identification of the nutritional content of foods [28], especially when the labels include colors and familiar symbols [19, 22]. However, some have reported a weaker impact of labels on attention and consumption [8].

Research studies show inconsistent results regarding the most effective type of label [15, 28]. Some favor graded summary labels (e.g., Nutri-Score) but note that this depends on the outcome measure and setting which makes the studies not comparable [28]. Others advocate for warning labels, graded labels, and reductive labels in that order [22].

Attention to Nutrition Facts labels depends on the type of labels. Some studies show that interpretive labels shift attention away [8], while others say they improve the search for nutritional information more than reductive labels [28]. Attention to single summary logos is faster but can lead to incorrect evaluations, and consumers may not notice when such logos are absent [28].

Healthfulness evaluations of products are higher for reductive and interpretive labels of unhealthy products. However, interpretative nutrient-specific labels also work for healthier products [8]. Healthy identification is better for products with summary labels than nutrient-specific labels, but both are effective [8]. Tastiness evaluations are lower for products with interpretative labels, suggesting that healthy foods may be perceived as not tasty [8]. Regarding the food products, the presence of reference information, financial incentives, and health risk information also impacts consumer behavior related to FOP labels [26].

Including financial incentives may be more effective than merely presenting information, as seen with FOP labels that include reference information. Other situational factors are also relevant, including familiarity [13], healthy eating prompts, social norm messages, presentation order of labels [26], salient health goal reminders [22], and time pressure [31].

It is worth noting that most research has been conducted in artificial environments. Typically, the subjects view the labels on a computer or as photographs in a research facility rather than in a real supermarket [7, 28, 32]. While these experimental studies commonly observe improvements in food choices, evidence suggests that the impact of FOP labels is far weaker in real-life studies. Their impact on long-term diet or consumption is very different from that of a one-time choice [32]. It is clear that there is a need for more research on variables that may increase the effectiveness of FOP food labels on eating, in real purchase settings, or investigating novel FOP food labeling.

Digital Technologies and Front-of-Package Food Labels

Digital technologies can further support FOP food labeling in helping consumers choose or consume healthier foods [26]. They can provide consumers with information about FOP labels, in combination with other aspects of food products or situational factors. This is typically done in point-of-purchase settings, including online grocery stores, quick-response codes, smartphone apps, digital touchscreens, self-checkout scanning, and video carts [33–35]. For instance, FOP labels may be presented based on the entire basket of products as well as product nutritional data, in combination with food swaps. This can be done in relation to purchases by other consumers or personalized dietary needs.

Regarding labeling the entire basket, Shin et al. [36] investigated whether purchase behavior was impacted by dynamic and real-time basket feedback of consumer products in terms of aggregated Nutri-Scores, physical activity equivalents, and daily recommended intake of nutrients. Additionally, consumers could also sort and review their purchases at the checkout. They found that the intervention increased the weighted Nutri-Score and reduced the sugar content of the purchased foods. Fuchs et al. [37] investigated the possible value of providing Nutri-Score labeling of individual products. They found that participants then chose products with higher nutritional quality.

Food swaps are another application of digital technologies. With this strategy, recommendations for healthier product options are made after consumers have selected the products. For example, De Bauw et al. [38] investigated how the selection of products is influenced by Nutri-Score and eco-labeling at both the individual product and basket levels, other consumers' product selection, and product recommendation agents. They found that nutritional quality was higher when individual products were labeled. However, basket scores, social norms, and recommendation agents did not shift the initial selections.

Another strategy is the provision of personalized information to consumers. Fuchs et al. [39] presented combined tailored food labels based on user-specific dietary needs using a smartphone app. They found that participants were more likely to recommend the app to their friends, that it helped them assess their dietary intake, and that it presented relevant recommendations based on their lifestyle, more so than standard labels. Similarly, Ljusic et al. [27] investigated digitalized FOP food labels that presented static labels through a digital medium, interactive labels with the option of more information, and technology-enabled labels based on personalized, dynamic, and real-time information on consumers' behavior. Compared to static labels, interactive labels had a lesser impact, while technology-enabled labels had a greater impact on consumer behavior.

Conclusions

This chapter has presented the key characteristics of FOP labels. They can be classified as interpretative or reductive nutrient-specific. The former explicitly states the healthfulness of the food, while the latter focuses on the content of nutrients in the food. Interpretive labels may present information as a single value (e.g., a tick is present or absent) or as a graded value (e.g., A to E lettering in Nutri-Score). Similarly, nutrient-specific labels may take the form of a single value (e.g., a warning label indicating that the food has a high salt content) or as a graded value (e.g., Multiple Traffic Lights indicating that the level of nutrients is high, medium, or low) and often also include numerical values (e.g., amount of salt per serving).

There has been an increase in mandatory labels worldwide and a shift from single summary labels (e.g., a tick) to graded summary labels (e.g., Nutri-Score) in Europe, and more warning labels in the Americas.

FOP labels impact consumer behavior and differ in terms of purchase, consumption, attention, and subjective measures. Overall, interpretive labels are more helpful than reductive labels. Graded summary and warning labels are promising but have less impact in real-life settings.

One promising label type is the graded summary system such as Nutri-Score. Their advantages include providing simple information to consumers, a single evaluation rather than multiple evaluations [8, 22], more nuanced information than single summary labels, and being more adaptable to changes in labeling requirements without causing confusion.

Additionally, the food industry may be more positive towards this type of label than warning labels. The challenges with current summary labels are that they may not include all nutrients and their synergies, and that a single worldwide labeling algorithm may not meet the needs of many individuals [18]. The flaws with nutrient-specific labels, such as Multiple Traffic Lights, are that evaluating the healthfulness of the quantities of different nutrients can be misleading and may increase consumer effort or lead to confusion, especially when countries have different national dietary guidelines.

Digital technologies can support FOP labels by presenting valuable information such as product nutritional data, a summary of the entire basket, purchases by other consumers, personalized dietary needs, or by combining food swaps.

In conclusion, FOP labels hold much promise for helping consumers select a healthier diet. For that reason, FOP labels are potentially a valuable tool for health promotion. However, there is still much uncertainty regarding which design is most effective and the extent to which FOP labels have a positive impact on population diets when used in real-world situations such as supermarkets.

References

1. World Health Organization. Obesity and overweight. 2025. https://www.who.int/news-room/fact-sheets/detail/obesity-and-overweight. Accessed 7 Oct 2025.
2. World Health Organization. The challenge of obesity. 2024. https://www.who.int/europe/news-room/fact-sheets/item/the-challenge-of-obesity. Accessed 7 Oct 2025.
3. Bremner JD, Moazzami K, Wittbrodt MT, Nye JA, Lima BB, Gillespie CF, et al. Diet, stress and mental health. Nutrients. 2020;12:2428.
4. Popkin BM, Barquera S, Corvalan C, Hofman KJ, Monteiro C, Ng SW, et al. Towards unified and impactful policies to reduce ultra-processed food consumption and promote healthier eating. Lancet Diab Endocrinol. 2021;9:462–70.
5. Forray AI, Borzan CA. Implementation of national nutrition policies and strategies to reduce unhealthy diets: an ecological analysis of 194 countries from 2017 to 2021. Nutrients. 2024;16:911.
6. Alsubhi M, Blake M, Nguyen T, Majmudar I, Moodie M, Ananthapavan J. Consumer willingness to pay for healthier food products: a systematic review. Obes Rev. 2023;24:e13525.
7. Temple NJ. Front-of-package food labels: a narrative review. Appetite. 2020;144:104485.
8. Ikonen I, Sotgiu S, Aydinli A, Verlegh PWJ. Consumer effects of front-of-package nutrition labeling: An interdisciplinary meta-analysis. J Acad Market Sci. 2020;48:360–83.
9. U.S. Food and Drug Administration. What's on the Nutrition Facts Label. 2024. https://www.fda.gov/food/nutrition-facts-label/whats-nutrition-facts-label. Accessed 26 Oct 2025.
10. Swedish Food Agency. The Nordic Keyhole scheme. 2018. https://food.ec.europa.eu/system/files/2018-04/comm_ahac_20180423_pres2.pdf. Accessed 21 Nov 2025.
11. Kanter R, Vanderlee L, Vandevijvere S. Front-of-package nutrition labelling policy: global progress and future directions. Public Health Nutr. 2018;21:1399–408.
12. Jones A, Neal B, Reeve B, Mhurch CN, Thow AM. Front-of-pack nutrition labelling to promote healthier diets: current practice and opportunities to strengthen regulation worldwide. BMJ Glob Health. 2019;4:e001882.
13. Batista MF, de Carvalho-Ferreira JP, Thimoteo da Cunha D, De Rosso VV. Front-of-package nutrition labeling as a driver for healthier food choices: lessons learned and future perspectives. Compr Rev Food Sci Food Saf. 2023;22:535–86.
14. Afroza U, Abrar AK, Nowar A, Sobhan S, Mohammad M, Ide N, et al. Global overview of government-endorsed nutrition labeling policies of packaged foods: a document review. Front Public Health. 2024;12:1426639.
15. An R, Shi Y, Shen J, Bullard T, Liu G, Yang Q, et al. Effect of front-of-package nutrition labeling on food purchases: a systematic review. Public Health. 2021;191:59–67.
16. World Health Organization. Guiding principles and framework manual for front-of-pack labelling for promoting healthy diet. 2019. https://cdn.who.int/media/docs/default-source/healthy-diet/guidingprinciples-labelling-promoting-healthydiet.pdf?sfvrsn=65e3a8c1_7&download=true. Accessed 7 Oct 2024.

17. Storcksdieck Genannt Bonsmann S, Marandola G, Ciriolo E, Van Bavel R, Wollgast J. Front-of-pack nutrition labelling schemes: a comprehensive review, EUR 29811 EN. Luxembourg: Publications Office of the European Union; 2020.
18. Donini LM, Berry EM, Folkvord F, Jansen L, Leroy F, Şimşek O, et al. Front-of-pack labels: "directive" versus "informative" approaches. Nutrition. 2023;105:111861.
19. Hersey JC, Wohlgenant KC, Arsenault JE, Kosa KM, Muth MK. Effects of front-of-package and shelf nutrition labeling systems on consumers. Nutr Rev. 2013;71:1–14.
20. Cebas. Nutri Score European nutrition label for stock photo. 2025. Istockphoto.com/Cebas. https://www.istockphoto.com/photo/nutri-score-european-nutrition-label-for-food-gm2205746503-623119200?clarity=false. Accessed 26 Oct 2025.
21. U.S. Food and Drug Administration. FDA issues proposed rule on front-of-package nutrition labeling. 2025. https://www.fda.gov/food/hfp-constituent-updates/fda-issues-proposed-rule-front-package-nutrition-labeling. Accessed 26 Oct 2025.
22. Roberto CA, Ng SW, Ganderats-Fuentes M, Hammond D, Barquera S, Jauregui A, Taillie LS. The influence of front-of-package nutrition labeling on consumer behavior and product reformulation. Ann Rev Nutr. 2021;41:529–50.
23. Temple NJ. Fat, sugar, whole grains and heart disease: 50 years of confusion. Nutrients. 2018;10:39.
24. Zhen C, Zheng X. The impact of NuVal shelf nutrition labels on food purchase. Appl Econ Perspect Policy. 2020;42:870–87.
25. Holbrook MB. What is consumer research? J Consum Res. 1987;14:128–32.
26. Schruff-Lim E-M, Van Loo EJ, can Kleef E, van Trijp HCM. Turning FOP nutrition labels into action: a systematic review of label+ interventions. Food Policy. 2023;120:102479.
27. Ljusic N, Fagerstrøm A, Pawar S, Arntzen E. Effects of digitalized front-of-package food labels on healthy food-related behavior: a systematic review. Behav Sci. 2022;12:363.
28. Kelly B, Vanderlee L, Vandevijvere S. The potential effectiveness of front-of-pack nutrition labeling for improving population diets. Ann Rev Nutr. 2024;44:1399–408.
29. Jin H, Li Y, Li D, Zheng J. The effects of physical activity calorie equivalent labeling on dieters' food consumption and post-consumption physical activity. J Consum Aff. 2020;54:723–41.
30. Taillie LS, Hall MG, Popkin BM, Ng SW, Murukutla N. Experimental studies of front-of-package nutrient warning labels on sugar-sweetened beverages and ultra-processed foods: a scoping review. Nutrients. 2020;12:569.
31. Sanjari SS, Jahn S, Boztug Y. Dual-process theory and consumer response to front-of-package nutrition label formats. Nutr Rev. 2017;75:871–82.
32. Muzzioli L, Scenna D, Frigerio F, Manuela S, Poggiogalle E, Giusti AA, et al. Nutri-Score effectiveness in improving consumers' nutrition literacy, food choices, health, and healthy eating pattern adherence: a systematic review. Nutrition. 2025;140:112880.
33. Granheim SI, Løvhaug AL, Terragni L, Torheim LE, Thurston M. Mapping the digital food environment: a systematic scoping review. Obesity Rev. 2022;23:e13356.
34. Inman JJ, Nikolova H. Shopper-facing retail technology: a retailer adoption decision framework incorporating shopper attitudes and privacy concerns. J Retail. 2017;93:7–28.
35. Werle COC, Nohlen HU, Pantazi M. Literature review on means of food information provision other than packaging labels. Luxembourg: Publications Office of the European Union; 2022.
36. Shin S, van Dam RM, Finkelstein EA. The effect of dynamic food labels with real-time feedback on diet quality: results from a randomized controlled trial. Nutrients. 2020;12:2158.
37. Fuchs KL, Lian J, Michels L, Mayer S, Toniato E, Tiefenback V. Effects of digital food labels on healthy food choices in online grocery shopping. Nutrients. 2022;14:2044.
38. De Bauw M, De La Revilla LS, Poppe V, Matthys C, Vranken L. Digital nudges to stimulate healthy and pro-environmental food choices in E-groceries. Appetite. 2022;172:105971.
39. Fuchs K, Barattin T, Haldimann M, Ilic A. Towards tailoring digital food labels: Insights of a smart-RCT on user-specific interpretation of food composition data. In: Proceedings of the 5th international workshop on multimedia assisted dietary management. 2019.

Genomics Medicine and Personalized Nutrition

11

Ashwini Rajasekaran, Jasmine Chen, and Karen Davison

Abstract

- Genomic medicine integrates individual genomic information as part of one's health care. Nutrigenetics and nutrigenomics are related fields that target genes, diet, and health.
- Nutrigenetics focuses on the interactions of the inherited genome and nutrition.
- Nutrigenomics encompasses genome-based patterns such as DNA methylation, epigenetics, and metabolic regulation influenced by nutritional uptake.
- Genomic-based personalized nutrition (GBPN) integrates genetic, phenotypic, and comprehensive nutrition assessment data to provide precise dietary guidance to help optimize health status.
- Despite steady development in GBPN, there is continued need for robust scientific evidence that considers multifactorial disease etiology, genomic diversity, as well as ethical, legal, policy, and system infrastructure considerations.

A. Rajasekaran
Centre for Heart Lung Innovation, University of British Columbia and St. Paul's Hospital, Vancouver, BC, Canada

J. Chen
Department of Public Health and Social Policy, University of Victoria, Victoria, BC, Canada
e-mail: jaschen@uvic.ca

K. Davison (✉)
Institute for Life Course and Aging, University of Toronto & The Centre of Clinical Excellence, Toronto, ON, Canada

Centre for Science, Athabasca University, Athabasca, AB, Canada
e-mail: karend@athabascau.ca

N. J. Temple, T. Wilson (eds.), *Pocket Primer for Nutritional Health*,
https://doi.org/10.1007/978-3-032-25402-3_11

Introduction: Genome-Based Personalized Nutrition

Nutrition and genetic interactions are important determinants of human health. It is estimated that genetic predisposition accounts for 20–30% of health outcomes related to premature mortality [1]. Suboptimal diet is a major modifiable risk factor that contributes to chronic diseases of lifestyle (CDL) morbidity and mortality [2]. For some conditions, such as celiac disease, where dietary intervention circumvents metabolic deficiency, this is very well understood [3]. The potential of bioactive compounds to affect processes such as epigenetics and genomic imprinting [4] also demonstrates the relevance of nutrition and genetic interactions in the prevention and management of CDL.

Genomic-based personalized nutrition (GBPN) is based on the complementary fields of nutrigenetics and nutrigenomics [4]. Nutrigenetics considers the effects of inter-individual differences of genetic variants on responses to nutrients and other bioactive food components in relation to health and disease. Conversely, nutrigenomics considers the effect of nutrition-related DNA modifications and regulatory interactions of nutrients and bioactive food components with DNA and RNA elements and understanding the physiological responses to specific diets. It explains how dietary components affect gene expression resulting in gain or loss of function of those proteins. Nutritional genomics, which encompasses nutrigenomics and nutrigenetics, focuses on the interactions between gene and dietary components.

Nutriepigenetics specifically focuses on how dietary components influence epigenetic modifications, which are changes in gene expression that do not alter the DNA sequence [5]. Unlike the DNA sequence, epigenetic marks can undergo changes in response to several stimuli including nutrition exposures. Epigenetic dysregulation due to dietary deficiencies or excesses may affect gene expression and impact genome stability by causing mutations in the DNA sequence or chromosomal instability resulting in abnormal gene dosage and adverse phenotypes such as CDL [6].

The underlying goals of GBPN are to translate information from genetic tests into tailored nutrition recommendations to prevent or manage specific health outcomes. It may be used along with other data such as socioeconomics, lifestyle habits, life stage, individual and family health history, and various biochemical indicators including gut microbiome composition. These practices, considered as a part of precision or personalized medicine, are intended to customize healthcare to individuals and subgroups.

Gene-Diet Interactions: Translating Research to Practice

A Brief Overview

Every human genome has more than 3 million single-nucleotide variants compared to ~3 billion base pairs in the reference genome; about 1% of a person's genome varies from the reference sequence [7]. This genetic variation accounts for differences in characteristics such as physical traits, disease susceptibility, drug responses, and nutrient metabolism. Genetic variability arises from four major types of genomic variation. The first, and most extensively studied, is single-nucleotide polymorphisms (SNPs). These involve single base pair changes that may alter gene function. The second type are insertions and deletions (INDELs), which are short DNA fragment changes that can disrupt coding sequences or regulatory elements. The third type are copy number variants (CNVs), where segments of DNA, including entire genes, may be duplicated or deleted, resulting in variable copy numbers/gene dosage across individuals. The last are structural variants (SVs); these encompass larger genomic rearrangements such as translocations, inversions, and duplications, which can significantly alter genome architecture. Distribution of genetic variants varies across populations, with rare variants often showing strong geographic differentiation, influenced by factors such as evolutionary conservation, coding consequence, and negative selection [7].

Several dietary components interact with genetic variants and influence nutrient metabolism (Fig. 11.1) [8]. These interactions affect the expression of metabolism-associated genes, levels of expression or activities of enzymes that synthesize or catabolize a nutrient, amounts of bioactive nutrient products and their metabolites, and phenotypic outcomes such as CDL. These interactions can also be modulated by other factors, including microbiome composition, lifestyle, and epigenetic regulation.

Gene–diet interactions can induce epigenetic alterations including DNA methylation, histone modifications, and non-coding RNA activity that influence biological processes such as nutrient metabolism [9]. Nutritional transcriptomics can help identify genes and pathways that alter pre-disease states and assist in characterizing bioactive food components or nutrient-regulated pathways [10]. Nutritional proteomics helps to reveal how specific nutrients regulate protein expression and function. Nutritional metabolomics helps identify the metabolic shifts caused by specific nutrients or diets, and how nutrients interact with genetic and environmental stressors [5]. GBPN integrates multiomic profiling (genomics, proteomics, metabolomics, transcriptomics) in order to tailor dietary interventions according to biological needs.

Genomics and Nutrition Research

Several types of research inform GBPN practice. Genome-wide association studies (GWAS) and epigenome-wide association studies (EWAS) help identify genomic regions that are pertinent to complex traits such as BMI, fasting glucose, and fasting insulin [10]. GWAS examine SNPs across large populations to identify causal genetic variants. SNPs may influence metabolic pathways by altering enzyme activity or transporter function and affect nutrient absorption, digestion, transport, and excretion. EWAS examine genome-wide sets of epigenetic marks, such as DNA methylation, that are associated with a trait. Mendelian randomization, a method which uses genetic variants that are robustly associated with modifiable exposures, such as diet, may be used in GWAS and EWAS to explore causal links.

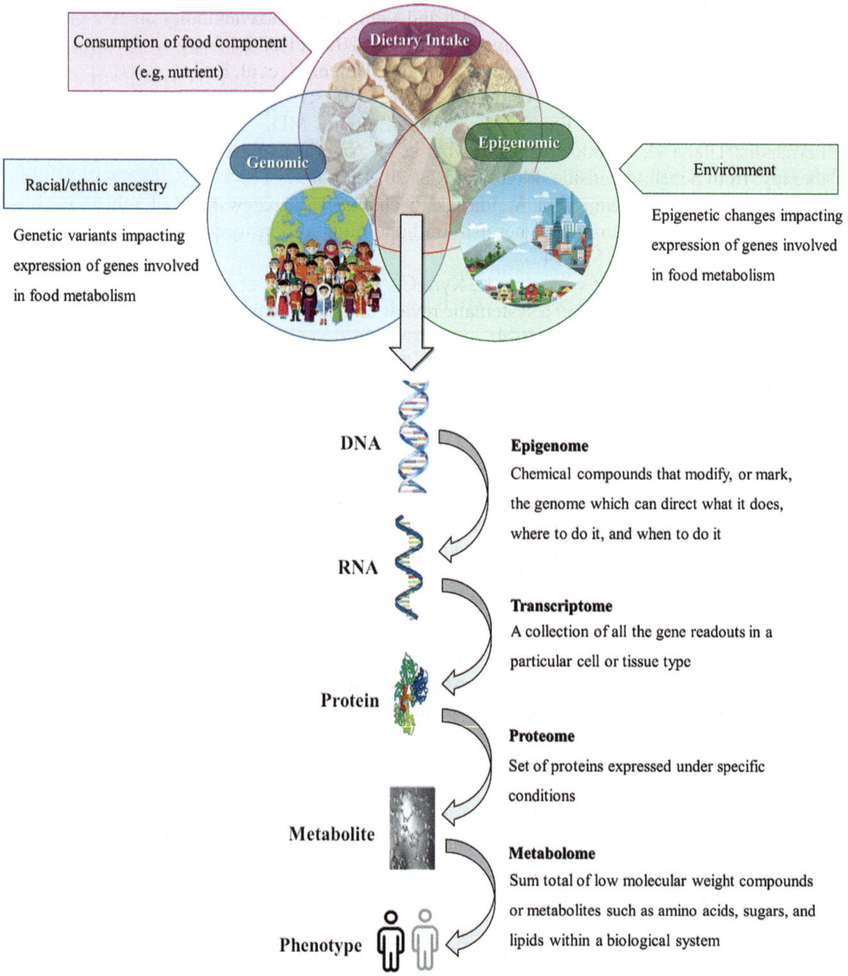

Fig. 11.1 Gene and diet interactions. (Adapted from Mullins et al. [8])

GBPN also integrates insights from epigenomics (e.g., DNA methylation, histone modifications) and transcriptomics (e.g., RNA-seq profiling of nutrient-responsive genes). GBPN strategies increasingly incorporate metabolomic and microbiome data to tailor interventions to individual biological contexts [11]. For example, dietary interventions that emphasize whole grains, vegetables, fruits, and lower intake of total and saturated fats have been shown to reduce risk among individuals with higher genetic risk scores of obesity [12]. Emerging technologies like 3D genome mapping examine how chromatin loops (i.e., structures in the genome that facilitate interactions between genomic regions) and topologically associated domains (i.e., self-interacting genomic regions) regulate gene expression and contribute to long-range epigenetic control [13]. Advances in epigenetic enzyme engineering are improving specificity while epigenetic signatures are being developed as non-invasive biomarkers for disease progression and treatment response [14].

Genomic-Based Personalized Nutrition

Applications and Testing

Many laboratory techniques have been developed to support GBPN, including mass spectrometry, infrared, atomic, ultraviolet, visible light, and magnetic resonance spectroscopy, chromatography, electrophoresis, microarrays, nuclear magnetic resonance, and bioinformatics [14]. These underpin omics technologies that enable identification of disease risk and the development of targeted assays. These assays span proteomics, lipidomics, metabolomics, and analysis of bioactive substances in food. Additional considerations include the development of functional foods and genetic products.

Molecular biology technologies are employed to detect SNPs and to identify candidate genes and polymorphisms involved in gene and nutrition-interactions. In health practice, variables that are typically examined include SNPs, candidate genes, and polymorphisms related to nutrient transport and metabolism, toxin elimination, oxidative stress protection, taste perception, food intolerances and sensitivities, body composition and weight management, eating habits, hormone metabolism, methylation, and physical activity responses. As with most scientific and technological domains, the global application of GBPN varies widely.

In vitro laboratory tests are frequently used to generate personalized insights for individuals who participate in GBPN. Different types of direct-to-consumer (DTC) genetic tests have been developed to assess predisposition to various health conditions. Companies such as 23andMe have received FDA authorization to market DTC genetic tests, including reports on carrier status, wellness, traits, and ancestry. These companies specify that their tests are not intended to diagnose medical conditions or provide dietary advice [15]. Some examples of nutrition-related components included in GBPN are highlighted in Table 11.1.

Genetic Testing and Dietary Guidance

The main concern about DTC genetic tests is that they are not regulated. Consumers can easily access them which raises issues about privacy and protection of genetic data. Some companies offer services without the direct involvement of health professionals. This can limit the consumer's interpretation of results and lead to psychological distress if they overestimate disease risk [15]. Computer-tailored nutrition education, based on artificial intelligence (AI) applications, may be used but the information may be clinically ambiguous [16]. From an ethical perspective, the information disseminated must be in accordance with the ability of the individual to properly understand and utilize it [17]. Any result based on insufficient

Table 11.1 Select examples of genetic polymorphisms, their related genes, dietary factors, and health outcome risks

Gene	Polymorphism	Dietary variable	Health outcome risk
ACE	Insertion/deletion (I/D)	Salt sensitivity	Type 2 diabetes (T2D) Hypertension
CYP1A2	A > C	Reduced ability to metabolize caffeine	Heart disease
CYP2R1	rs10741657 rs10766197	Increased need for food rich in vitamin D and for sun exposure	Lower vitamin D levels
FTO	rs9939609	Altered macronutrient metabolism	T2D, obesity
	rs1558902	Impact on weight loss, level of insulin, and HOMA-IR	Obesity
FUT2	rs602662 Gly258Ser	Increased need for food rich in vitamin B12	Lower vitamin B12 levels
GSTT1	Insertion/deletion (I/D)	Free radical production	Serum vitamin C deficiency
MTHFR	rs1801133 C677T A1298C A222V	High level of homocysteine Increased need for folic acid Altered macronutrient metabolism	Breast cancer, homocystinuria, cardiovascular disease, T2D, neural tube defects
NOS3	rs1799983	Altered macronutrient metabolism	Lipid metabolism disturbances
TAS1R2	rs35874116 Ile191Val	Altered carbohydrate responsiveness	Hypertriglyceridemia

Adapted from Naureen et al. [5]

evidence may lead to unnecessary clinical investigations and inappropriate use of resources.

GBPN practice must be based on clinically and empirically validated tests. Consumers need to work closely with a regulated health professional trained in GBPN who can assess whether the lab performing the test is accredited and if the results are clinically relevant. These professionals facilitate appropriate interventions (Fig. 11.2) which allow for a thorough consenting process, discussion about the nature and utility of the genetic tests, scope of the results, possible risks, and information concerning confidentiality. The success of GBPN largely depends on individual motivation and their perceptions about future benefits offered by such dietary changes [18].

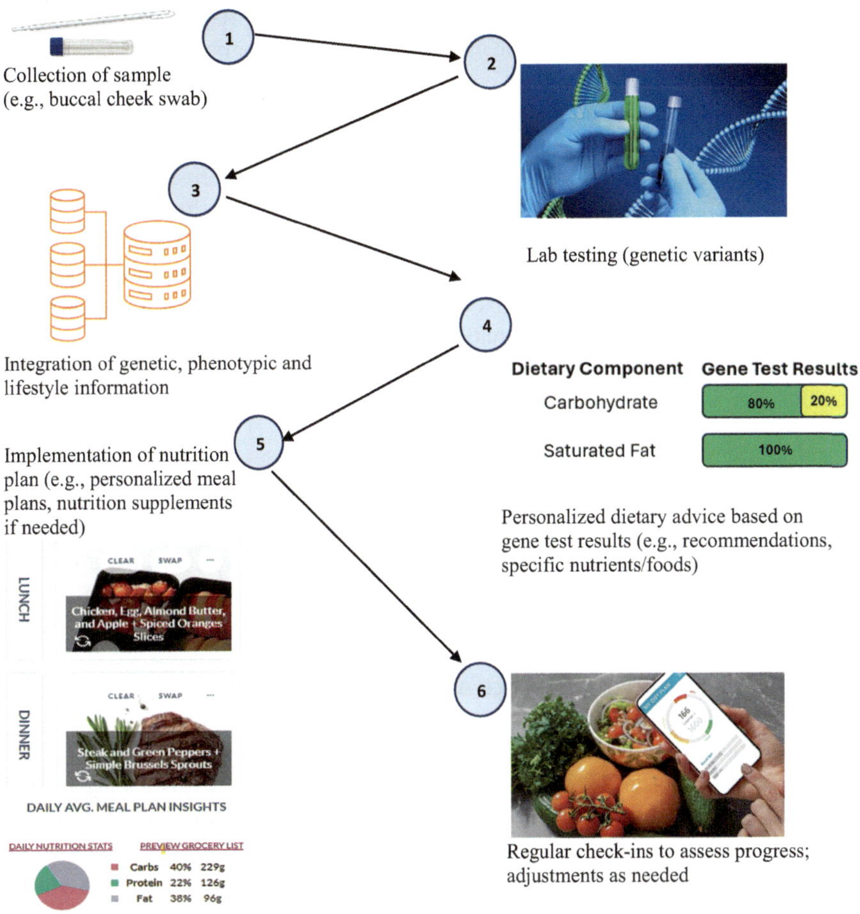

Fig. 11.2 Steps involved in GBPN practice

Genomic-Based Personalized Nutrition: Evidence and Progress

Emerging evidence suggests that GBPN may outperform population-based dietary recommendations for improving compliance and health outcomes [17–22]. Several studies report modest dietary improvements including fruit and vegetable consumption and decreased intake of red meat, salt, and saturated fat. In a 6-month RCT which examined changes in discretionary food and beverage intake between groups which either received GBPN guidance or general dietary advice [22], the intervention group had significantly lower intake of sugar, energy, total fat, saturated fat, and salt from discretionary items.

GBPN applications may be beneficial for long-term weight control. Dietary patterns emphasizing whole grains, vegetables, and fruit while limiting total and saturated fat have demonstrated the potential to lower the risk of carrying excess weight for people with high genetic predisposition scores for obesity [21]. However, findings in this area have not been consistent.

A systematic review, published in 2022, summarized dietary, physical activity, and health outcome effects reported in nine moderate to high-quality RCTs that tested GBPN [23]. The findings did not point to consistent benefits. This may be due to factors such as a lack of investigations from regions other than North America and Europe or individuals with different diseases. Furthermore, the complex relationships among genes, interventions, and outcomes may not have been captured. Another possibility is that there was bias related to blinding of participants. RCTs conducted after the 2022 systematic review provide some additional insights [24–26]. Based on the presently available evidence, it is premature to draw firm conclusions.

Challenges of Gene-Based Personalized Nutrition

The challenges of GBPN include limitations in current science, research, and practice.

Limitations of Current Science and Research

Most genetic testing is performed using DNA microarrays ("SNP chip") that can detect several thousand SNPs at a given time. Limitations of this testing include potential for errors in SNP identification or imputation of an unobserved genotype, exclusion of rare variants, and lack of account for other types of genetic alterations across the genome. This results in an incomplete understanding of the functionality of identified genetic alterations and can impact clinical utility.

Because most CDL are multifactorial and multigenic, studies are needed that account for gene-gene and gene-diet interactions in order to provide specific nutrigenetic recommendation algorithms. Many studies of SNPs are based on modest-sized samples and/or people of European ancestry which limits generalizability. Dietary intake measurement tools (e.g., food frequency questionnaires) used in these studies may lack validity and reliability in their reflection of long-term intakes. For these reasons in order that future studies provide improved understanding of nutrition metabolism and requirements, they should focus on the whole genome, genetic algorithms known to impact metabolism, and improved quantification of dietary intake.

Although the use of genomic signatures to predict health outcomes has evolved substantially, the evidence which links them to reliable prognostic biomarkers remains limited [10]. Biomarkers, such as serum retinol, ferritin, insulin secretion, and blood glucose levels, have been used for diagnostics. However, there remains incomplete understanding of the genomic and non-genomic pathways of bioactive components and how they interact to impact health outcomes and a lack of key health biomarkers and signatures to define different optimal responses.

There is a need for study of the impact of dietary supplementation in GBPN [27]. For example, some subpopulations may derive more benefit from specific supplements such as omega-3 fatty acids [28, 29]. The utility of subgroup exploration is still debated. There is a clear need for rigorous measurement tools and statistical techniques to decipher effect modification [30].

Barriers in Practice

Personalized health approaches rely on shared decision making among consumers and multidisciplinary healthcare teams (e.g., physicians, geneticists, dietitians). These teams should include experts who can analyze genetic profiles, integrate data from omics analyses, and translate knowledge acquired into dietary recommendations and nutritional education. The actions by these teams are influenced by public policies and healthcare infrastructures.

The differences among policies, regulations, and evidence-informed system infrastructure to guide GBPN present risks for consumers. Some countries regulate the genetic testing industry; however, they are unable to control offshore companies that can access local markets via the internet. As a result, there are potential problems related to informed consent, privacy, scientific validity, and the provision of genetic findings without appropriate medical oversight. While health professionals may act as intermediaries between the genetic testing companies and consumers, few feel qualified to do so and often state that there are insufficient practice guidelines and educational resources [31]. Only a few health professional bodies formally recognize GBPN. The American Nutrition Association offers nutritional genomics training and certification. In addition, the Academy of Nutrition and Dietetics and the American Council on Exercise have formulated evidence-based practice guidelines that underscore the significance of customizing interventions that includes genetic information [32]. Clearly, the evidence that underlies GBPN needs to be as robust as that used for conventional nutritional guidelines. Fortunately, valuable tools are available including different frameworks to assess study quality, nature of the interactions (direct, intermediate, indirect relation to phenotype), nature of the genetic variant (causal link vs association), biological plausibility, and scientific validity [33]. In addition, care maps and clinical practice guidelines have been developed to guide professional practice [5].

To strengthen GBPN practice, appropriate evidence-informed policies and services should be based on ethical principles including autonomy, beneficence, justice, and minimization of psychological impact [33]. The high costs of comprehensive gene tests that include genome and exome sequencing and advisory services for interpretation of results limit GBPN practice and contribute to health disparities. Furthermore, consumers need to be assured that their genetic test results will not contribute to discrimination and impact their insurance coverage. In most jurisdictions, federal law prohibits health insurers from using genetic information to make decisions about whether to sell health insurance or how much to charge. But these rules may not apply to long-term care, life, or disability insurance.

Integrating Scientific and Technological Advancements

For GBPN tools to be truly meaningful, better integration with metagenomics is needed [34]. This includes incorporating knowledge about human physiology and metabolism. Also of importance, results from investigations of the intestinal microbial genome might improve diagnostics and interventions in GBPN. The human intestinal microbiome can be altered transiently by environmental factors, such as diet and medications, which can influence what is extracted from the diet and can also affect gene expression, protein synthesis, and the production of metabolites [35].

The fields of lipidomics, proteomics, and metabolomics continue to evolve; however, there are limits in the ability to encode metabolic paths and generate and apply biomarkers relevant to the development of dietary interventions [33]. The "exposome" research paradigm, which encompasses all accumulative environmental exposures in association with genetic factors, is recognized as a valid way in which to determine disease risk [33, 34]. The use of AI and machine learning/data-driven approaches may facilitate the integration of diverse genetic, metabolic, microbial, and clinical data allowing for predictive modeling of dietary responses. Wearable and mobile sensors to monitor nutritional status at the molecular level may offer non-invasive, real-time dietary information to support GBPN practice [35]. However, there are challenges in implementing these technologies in clinical and public health settings, including cost-effectiveness and the need to provide robust, reproducible, and interpretable results.

Conclusions

Research evidence has demonstrated that there are notable individual variations in nutrient metabolism and requirement. GBPN, including all omics technologies, may help provide more customized nutrition plans, enhance adherence, further clinical practice, and improve population health. However, the science and application of GBPN is still evolving, and challenges such as complexity, cost, and privacy concerns remain. There is a need for improved understanding in areas such as metagenomics and investigative paradigms that capture the complexity of gene-environment interactions in relation to disease etiology. Improvements in technologies, data interpretation tools, and practice resources will improve accuracy in results, produce robust evidence, and help ensure the practice standards are met. Health policy and law can play important roles in the formulation of ethical, professional practice, and legal regulations to ensure consistent, safe, and universal applications within an appropriate system infrastructure.

References

1. Kaplan RM, Milstein A. Contributions of health care to longevity: a review of 4 estimation methods. Ann Fam Med. 2019;17:267–72.
2. Melaku YA, Renzaho A, Gill TK, Taylor AW, Dal Grande E, de Courten B, et al. Burden and trend of diet-related non-communicable diseases in Australia and comparison with 34 OECD countries, 1990–2015: findings from the Global Burden of Disease Study 2015. Eur J Nutr. 2019;58:1299–313.
3. Abadie V, Han AS, Jabri B, Sollid LM. New insights on genes, gluten, and immunopathogenesis of celiac disease. Gastroenterology. 2024;167:4–22.
4. Divella R, Daniele A, Savino E, Paradiso A. Anticancer effects of nutraceuticals in the Mediterranean diet: an epigenetic diet model. Cancer Genom Proteom. 2020;17:335–50.
5. Naureen Z, Miggiano GAD, Aquilanti B, Velluti V, Matera G, Gagliardi L, et al. Genetic test for the prescription of diets in support of physical activity. Acta Biomed. 2020;91:e2020011.
6. Horne JR, Nielsen DE, Madill J, Robitaille J, Vohl MC, Mutch DM. Guiding global best practice in personalized nutrition based on genetics: the development of a nutrigenomics care map. J Acad Nutr Diet. 2022;122:259–69.
7. 1000 Genomes Project Consortium. An integrated map of genetic variation from 1,092 human genomes. Nature. 2012;491:56–65.
8. Mullins VA, Bresette W, Johnstone L, Hallmark B, Chilton FH. Genomics in personalized nutrition: can you "Eat for Your Genes"? Nutrients. 2020;12:3118.
9. Kiani AK, Bonetti G, Donato K, Kaftalli J, Herbst KL, Stuppia L, et al. Polymorphisms, diet and nutrigenomics. J Prev Med Hyg. 2022;63(2 Suppl 3):E125–41.
10. Battram T, Gaunt TR, Relton CL, Timpson NJ, Hemani G. A comparison of the genes and genesets identified by GWAS and EWAS of fifteen complex traits. Nat Commun. 2022;13:7816.
11. López de Maturana E, Alonso L, Alarcón P, Martín-Antoniano IA, Pineda S, Piorno L, et al. Challenges in the integration of omics and non-omics data. Genes. 2019;10:238.
12. Tan PY, Moore JB, Bai L, Tang G, Gong YY. In the context of the triple burden of malnutrition: a systematic review of gene-diet interactions and nutritional status. Crit Rev Food Sci Nutr. 2024;64:3235–63.
13. Trang KB, Pahl MC, Pippin JA, Su C, Littleton SH, Sharma P, et al. 3D genomic features across >50 diverse cell types reveal insights into the genomic architecture of childhood obesity. eLife. 2025;13:RP95411.
14. Park SH, Choi HK, Park JH, Hwang JT. Current insights into genome-based personalized nutrition technology: a patent review. Front Nutr. 2024;11:1346144.
15. Panacer KS. Ethical issues associated with direct-to-consumer genetic testing. Cureus. 2023;15:e39918.
16. Theodore Armand TP, Nfor KA, Kim JI, Kim HC. Applications of artificial intelligence, machine learning, and deep learning in nutrition: a systematic review. Nutrients. 2024;16:1073.
17. Nielsen DE, Shih S, El-Sohemy A. Perceptions of genetic testing for personalized nutrition: a randomized trial of DNA-based dietary advice. J Nutrigenet Nutrigenomics. 2014;7:94–104.
18. Araujo Almeida V, Littlejohn P, Cop I, Brown E, Afroze R, Davison KM. Comparison of nutrigenomics technology interface tools for consumers and health professionals: a sequential explanatory mixed methods investigation. J Med Internet Res. 2019;21:e12580.
19. Celis-Morales C, Livingstone KM, Marsaux CF, Macready AL, Fallaize R, O'Donovan CB, et al. On behalf of the Food4Me Study. Effect of personalized nutrition on health-related behaviour change: evidence from the Food4Me European randomized controlled trial. Int J Epidemiol. 2017;46:578–88.

20. Horne J, Gilliland J, O'Connor C, Seabrook J, Madill J. Enhanced long-term dietary change and adherence in a nutrigenomics-guided lifestyle intervention compared to a population-based (GLB/DPP) lifestyle intervention for weight management: results from the NOW randomised controlled trial. BMJ Nutr Prev Health. 2020;3:49–59.
21. Nielsen DE, Carere DA, Wang C, Roberts JS, Green RC, PGen Study Group. Diet and exercise changes following direct-to-consumer personal genomic testing. BMC Med Genom. 2017;10:24.
22. Livingstone KM, Celis-Morales C, Navas-Carretero S, San-Cristobal R, Forster H, Woolhead C, et al. Personalised nutrition advice reduces intake of discretionary foods and beverages: findings from the Food4Me randomised controlled trial. Int J Behav Nutr Phys Act. 2021;18:70.
23. Shyam S, Lee KX, Tan ASW, Khoo TA, Harikrishnan S, Lalani SA, et al. Effect of personalized nutrition on dietary, physical activity, and health outcomes: a systematic review of randomized trials. Nutrients. 2022;14:4104.
24. Wong O, Marshall K, Sicova M, Guest NS, García-Bailo B, El-Sohemy A. CYP1A2 genotype modifies the effects of caffeine compared with placebo on muscle strength in competitive male athletes. Int J Sport Nutr Exerc Metab. 2021;31:420–6.
25. Lee GY, Lee J, Kim JH, Chung KM, Han SN. Impact of recognition of genetic information related to BMI on changes in physical activity, dietary intake, and blood cholesterol level: a randomized controlled trial. Eur J Nutr. 2025;64:190.
26. Galmés S, Palou-March A, Pigsborg K, Adnan Aldubayane M, Gormseng SMO, Callejah A, et al. Personalized nutrition to mitigate inflammation in genetically predisposed individuals: a secondary analysis of the Danish PREVENTOMICS intervention. Food Sci Human Wellness. 2025;14:9250318.
27. Hill A, Starchl C, Dresen E, Stoppe C, Amrein K. An update of the effects of vitamins D and C in critical illness. Front Med. 2023;9:1083760.
28. Coates PM, Bailey RL, Blumberg JB, El-Sohemy A, Floyd E, Goldenberg JZ, et al. The evolution of science and regulation of dietary supplements: past, present, and future. J Nutr. 2024;154:2335–45.
29. Manson JE, Bassuk SS, Cook NR, Lee IM, Mora S, Albert CM, et al. VITAL Research Group. Vitamin D, marine n-3 fatty acids, and primary prevention of cardiovascular disease current evidence. Circ Res. 2020;126:112–28.
30. Keathley J, Garneau V, Marcil V, Mutch DM, Robitaille J, Rudkowska I, et al. Clinical practice guidelines using GRADE and AGREE II for the impact of genetic variants on plasma lipid/lipoprotein/apolipoprotein responsiveness to omega-3 fatty acids. Front Nutr. 2022;8:768474.
31. Roosan D, Wu Y, Tran M, Huang Y, Baskys A, Roosan MR. Opportunities to integrate nutrigenomics into clinical practice and patient counseling. Eur J Clin Nutr. 2023;77:36–44.
32. Robinson J, Nitschke E, Tovar A, Mattar L, Gottesman K, Hamlett P, et al. Nutrition and physical activity interventions provided by nutrition and exercise practitioners for the general population: an evidence-based practice guideline from the Academy of Nutrition and Dietetics and American Council on Exercise. J Acad Nutr Diet. 2023;123:1215–37.
33. Singar S, Nagpal R, Arjmandi BH, Akhavan NS. Personalized nutrition: tailoring dietary recommendations through genetic insights. Nutrients. 2024;16:2673.
34. Lampe JW, Navarro SL, Hullar MA, Shojaie A. Inter-individual differences in response to dietary intervention: integrating omics platforms towards personalised dietary recommendations. Proc Nutr Soc. 2013;72:207–18.
35. Sempionatto JR, Montiel VR-V, Vargas E, Teymourian H, Wang J. Wearable and mobile sensors for personalized nutrition. ACS Sens. 2021;6:1745–60.

Nutritional Health and the Microbiome 12

Allison L. Brichacek, Katherine A. Maki, and Nicole Farmer

Abstract

- The human gut microbiome is both an ecosystem and a functional partner in nutrition.
- Features of the microbiome most relevant to diet, including diversity, resilience, and host factors, shape individual dietary responses.
- Microbial metabolism of carbohydrates, proteins, and fats generate signaling molecules through the diet–microbiome–metabolite axis.
- Macro- and micro-nutrients and phytochemicals modulate bacterial abundance.
- Metabolic and signaling mechanisms are connected to broader dietary patterns and food processing, and influence human health and chronic disease risk.

A. L. Brichacek (✉)
Department of Laboratory Medicine, National Institutes of Health Clinical Center, Bethesda, MD, USA
e-mail: allison.brichacek@nih.gov

K. A. Maki · N. Farmer
Translational Biobehavioral and Health Promotion Branch, National Institutes of Health Clinical Center, Bethesda, MD, USA
e-mail: katherine.maki@nih.gov; nicole.farmer@nih.gov

N. J. Temple, T. Wilson (eds.), *Pocket Primer for Nutritional Health*,
https://doi.org/10.1007/978-3-032-25402-3_12

Prokaryote Phyla Nomenclature

Updated name	Former name
Bacteroidota	Bacteroidetes
Bacillota	Firmicutes
Pseudomonadota	Proteobacteria
Actinomycetota	Actinobacteria
Verrucomicrobiota	Verrucomicrobia

Note: The International Code of Nomenclature of Prokaryotes (ICNP) voted to change the taxonomic nomenclature of phyla of prokaryotes in 2021 [1], and in 2023, the National Center for Biotechnology Information (NCBI) Taxonomy database adopted the inclusion of formalized ICNP nomenclature in their taxonomy browser entries [2, 3]. Prokaryote phylum names have been updated throughout this chapter to maintain consistency with ICNP and NCBI standards

Introduction

Over the past two decades, research on the gut microbiome and nutrition has evolved from cataloging microbial species to investigating how food and dietary components shape this complex ecosystem. The human gut *microbiota* is the diverse community of microorganisms inhabiting the gastrointestinal (GI) tract, including bacteria, archaea, eukaryotic fungi, protozoa, and viruses [4]. The term *microbiome* refers to this community of microorganisms along with the collective genomes and gene products of its members. While most current understanding of the gut microbiome centers on the abundance, diversity, and function of bacteria, researchers work to uncover the roles of the other resident microorganisms in shaping host physiology, immune function, and health outcomes.

For clinicians and scientists involved in the nutrition field, understanding how diet modulates the gut microbiome is of increasing relevance. Dietary factors, including nutrients, bioactive ingredients, food additives, and preparation or processing methods, can alter the composition and metabolic activity of the gut microbiome, with downstream host implications. Advances in sequencing, metabolomics, and computational modeling enable detailed exploration of these interactions. Substantial evidence indicates that the gut microbiome mediates many of the physiological effects of diet, including nutrient metabolism, energy balance, immune responses, intestinal barrier function, and inflammatory signaling pathways. Recognizing the microbiome as an intermediary between diet and health suggests new opportunities for targeted nutritional interventions aimed at optimizing microbiome–host interactions for improved health outcomes.

The Human Gut Microbiome: Ecosystem and Core Functions

Ecosystem

On average, the human body harbors 10^{13}–10^{14} bacterial cells, with the vast majority residing in the colon's low-oxygen environment. Contrary to earlier estimates suggesting bacteria outnumber human cells by a 10:1 ratio, current evidence indicates the numbers are about 1:1 [5]. Community composition of the adult gut microbiota is typically dominated by members of the phyla Bacteroidota and Bacillota, with additional functional contributions from Actinomycetota and Verrucomicrobiota [6]. Commonly observed genera in the colon include early colonizers like *Bifidobacterium*, *Lactobacillus*, and *Prevotella* [7], as well as key carbohydrate- and starch-degrading bacteria including *Akkermansia*, *Bacteroides*, *Faecalibacterium*, *Roseburia*, and *Ruminococcus* [6]. Each individual harbors a distinct gut microbial profile, shaped in part by host genetics, but driven more strongly by modifiable factors such as diet, environmental exposures, early-life events (including birth mode and infant feeding practices), medication use, and lifestyle patterns (see section "Host factors") [7].

General Biological Functions

Biosynthesis of Vitamins and Fatty Acids

The gut microbiota is essential for health and homeostasis, producing bioactive compounds that humans cannot synthesize in sufficient quantities. Studies using germ-free animals, which lack a gut microbiome, highlight the nutritional importance of GI bacteria. For example, germ-free animals raised in sterile conditions have significantly lower levels of short-chain fatty acids (SCFAs) in their colon and bloodstream, and need diets supplemented with vitamins B and K. Although dietary intake of phylloquinone (K_1) is the primary source of vitamin K, microbial production (K_2) may contribute up to 30–50% of daily vitamin K needs. In addition, many commensal bacteria possess de novo biosynthetic pathways for B vitamins [8]. Microbes that are efficient vitamin producers have specific properties to facilitate the import of precursor substrates and recycling of vitamin fragments for reuse. These features promote microbial self-sufficiency and enable vitamin sharing across the microbial community and with the host.

Dietary fibers and complex carbohydrates that escape digestion in the small intestine reach the colon, where gut microbes ferment them to produce SCFAs like acetate, butyrate, and propionate [9]. Fermentable fibers, including resistant starch, inulin, pectins, and β-glucans, are key dietary substrates for SCFA production [10]. When fiber intake is low, the microbiota can shift to fermenting host-derived mucin glycans, which help sustain SCFA production but may compromise GI barrier integrity [11]. Pyruvate is a central component of this fermentation process and is routed into different metabolic pathways depending on the microbial enzyme capacity and community energy needs. With some exceptions, acetate and propionate are produced largely by gram-negative Bacteroidota, while butyrate is primarily generated by gram-positive Bacillota. The physiologic roles of SCFAs in GI and systemic health are discussed in section "Short-chain fatty acids".

The identification of specialized epithelial transporters for bacterially derived vitamins and SCFAs in the large intestine underscores their importance for both colonocyte function and systemic metabolism. These transport processes highlight how the gut microbiome acts as a dynamic metabolic organ that integrates dietary inputs, microbial biosynthesis, and interspecies metabolite exchange to influence host micronutrient availability, SCFA profiles, and overall energy homeostasis.

Microbiome Characteristics Relevant to Diet

Diversity

High microbiota diversity, defined as the presence of many different bacterial species, is generally viewed as a marker of good gut health because it is usually associated with robust digestion, nutrient absorption, metabolite production, resilience to perturbations, and immune regulation [12]. For example, persons who consume a high amount of fermented foods have shown increased microbiome diversity and reduced inflammatory markers, while a high-fiber diet enhances microbial function and homeostatic immune responses [13]. Diets based on the Healthy Eating Index, including the Mediterranean diet, support greater microbial diversity and the generation of beneficial postbiotics [14]. However, high microbial diversity does not always translate to better health and has been associated with increased colonic transit time and higher systemic levels of potentially harmful protein-derived metabolites [15].

Resilience

The term "resilience" has been used by scientific disciplines, including engineering and ecological scientists, as the ability of a system to resist disturbances and remain stable. This is a controversial term in the microbiome field which defines resilience as the ability of microbial communities to return to their original state or resist change [16]. Some researchers claim that resilience and resistance are imperative characteristics of a healthy microbiota as these show the ability to stabilize, adapt, and recover from different stressors to maintain function [12, 17]. Factors that can affect the resilience of gut microbiota include microbial diversity, metabolic flexibility, functional redundancy, host-microbe and microbe-microbe interactions, and microbial products [18]. Interindividual differences may also drive microbial resilience, including the immune system, diet, physical activity, and mucus layer [18]. While for a healthy microbiota resilience is a benefit, this may prevent an unhealthy microbiota from being reshaped and help explain the failure of certain nutritional and therapeutic interventions [17].

Host Factors

The composition and function of the gut microbiome are affected by intrinsic and extrinsic factors, including host age, gender, genetics, immune system, chronic and metabolic diseases, region and environment, diet, lifestyle, and medications. Diet is one of the most significant factors that shapes the gut microbiome, as high-fat, high-sugar, and highly processed diets have been linked to gut dysbiosis [19]. Xenobiotics, chemical substances found in an organism that are not naturally occurring, can also be introduced with diet. While it is estimated that humans are exposed to 1–3 million xenobiotics during their lifetime, our diets contain >26,000 unique dietary xenobiotics, such as polyphenols, heavy metals, and food additives [20, 21]. Computational modeling to simulate diet-host-microbiome-disease interactions is under development and may provide more opportunities for personalized medicine [22].

Diet-Microbiome-Metabolite Axis

How Diet Shapes the Gut Metabolome

Gut microbiota can use non-digestible food components as substrates and generate chemical signals called metabolites which play important roles in regulating biological functions of the host. Host nutrient-sensing pathways in the gut, including sugar and fat-responsive enteroendocrine circuits, work together with microbiome-derived metabolites to signal the nutritional value of a meal and influence satiety, energy balance, and broader metabolic outcomes. Examining this diet-microbiome-metabolite axis is expected to deepen our understanding of how these interactions affect human health and may also partially explain individual variability in metabolism [23]. This section will discuss several of the metabolites most frequently measured in clinical trials.

Short-Chain Fatty Acids

SCFAs have been shown to exert beneficial effects on gut homeostasis and their deficiency has been associated with several disease states, including metabolic disease, cardiovascular disease (CVD), and colorectal cancer [24]. SCFAs are absorbed by the gut epithelium and metabolized into acetyl-CoA (acetate, butyrate) or transported to the liver to participate in gluconeogenesis (propionate) [24]. Because SCFA fermentation requires fiber availability, levels and composition are influenced by diet, and generally high-fiber or high-carbohydrate diets lead to higher SCFA production while diets higher in fat and/or protein tend to produce reduced levels of SCFAs [24] (Fig. 12.1). High-fiber diets promote the growth of SCFA-producing bacteria, such as *Bifidobacterium* and *Lactobacillus*, but this does not always translate to a significant increase in SCFAs [25].

Bile Acids

Primary BAs are synthesized in the liver and transported to the duodenum where select intestinal bacteria convert them into secondary BAs [26]. In humans, primary BAs are conjugated mainly with glycine, a modification that keeps BAs fully ionized at physiological pH and prevents them from disrupting bacterial membranes. Conversely, unconjugated BAs such as cholic acid and chenodeoxycholic acid have antimicrobial properties and can damage bacterial membranes [19]. BAs contribute

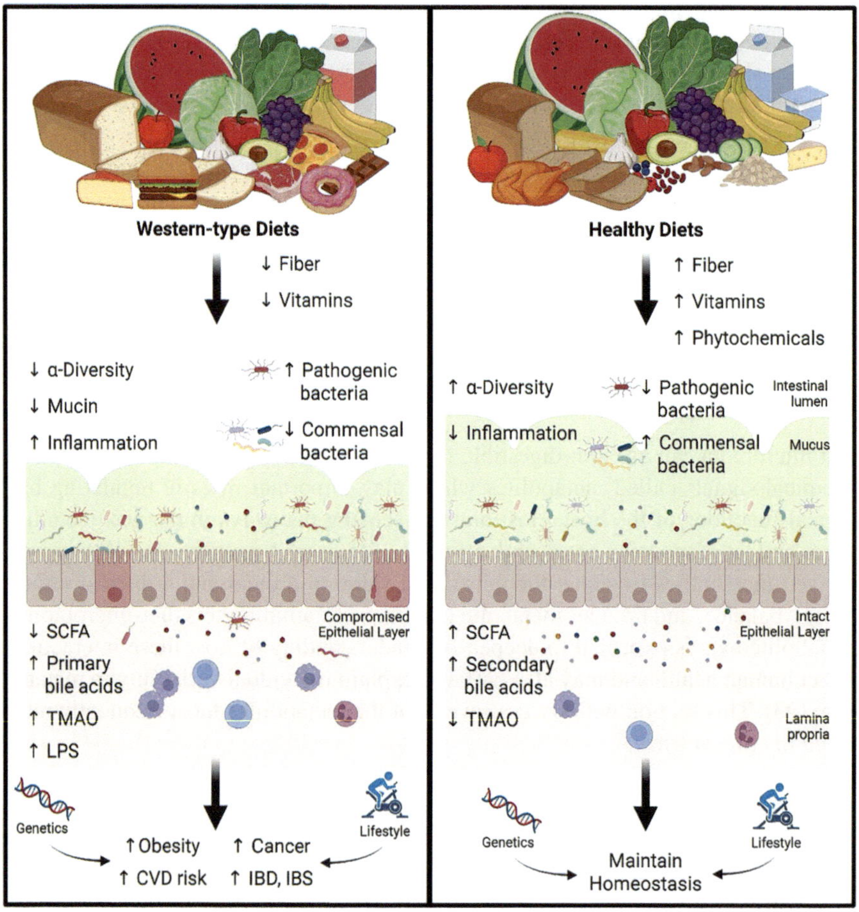

Fig. 12.1 Dietary patterns affect the gut microbiome and metabolites and are associated with risk of conditions and disease. Diet has been shown to highly impact the composition, structure, and function of the gut microbiome. In the left panel: Western-type diets, which typically have inadequate fiber and vitamin intake, result in reduced bacterial diversity and increased abundance of pathogenic bacteria. This lack of diversity and unbalanced proportions of bacteria lead to reduced production of SCFAs, reduced conjugation of bile acids (BAs), and increased systemic markers of consumed animal products (trimethylamine-*N*-oxide [TMAO]) and bacterial products (lipopolysaccharide [LPS]) outside of the gut due to weakened mucosal and epithelial barriers. Ultimately, the Western diet along with other host factors such as genetics and lifestyle may result in increased risk for obesity and various diseases. In the right panel: Healthy diets (e.g., Mediterranean-type diets, plant-based diets, etc.), which provide adequate fiber, vitamins, and other beneficial nutrients, have higher bacterial diversity and lower abundance of pathogenic bacteria compared to Western-type diets. Healthy diets promote gut microbiota that adequately produce SCFAs, conjugate primary into secondary BAs, and do not promote disease.

to intestinal barrier integrity, energy and metabolic regulation, immune function, and overall disease risk (Fig. 12.1) [26]. They also facilitate fat digestion and absorption in the small intestine and are linked to glucose and lipid homeostasis [27]. In animal models, Western-style diets increase BA production [28].

Amino Acids

Dietary and host-derived amino acids support microbial protein synthesis, but excess amino acids can be diverted into pathways that generate "uremic toxins". These metabolites can drive inflammation, activate the renin–angiotensin–aldosterone system, and disrupt cardiac and cellular function. L-carnitine and choline/phosphatidylcholine, abundant in animal products, are metabolized by microbial enzymes into trimethylamine (TMA) which is then converted in the liver to trimethylamine *N*-oxide (TMAO). TMAO influences lipid and glucose homeostasis, platelet activation, and tissue fibrosis; elevated levels have been associated with adverse outcomes in chronic kidney disease, type 2 diabetes, and CVD [29] (Fig. 12.1). Plant-based diets (i.e., vegetarian and vegan diets) are generally associated with improved cardiovascular outcomes compared with animal-based diets [30].

Postbiotics

Postbiotics, which are contents of inanimate microorganisms and/or their bioactive components that are beneficial to the host, are an emerging topic in nutritional and clinical studies. Postbiotics may be beneficial to the host due to the microbial metabolites or cellular components they induce. They may be safer than probiotics for populations such as newborns, the elderly, and patients with compromised immune systems because they are inactivated [31]. At present, postbiotics are mainly derived from traditional prebiotics, such as *Lactobacillus* spp., *Bifidobacterium* spp., *Bacteroides* spp., and *Akkermansia muciniphila* [31]. There are five mechanisms of action that have been proposed in relation to the benefits of postbiotics: (1) regulating the resident microbiota, (2) enhancing epithelial barrier functions, (3) regulating the local and systemic immune response, (4) modulating the systemic metabolic response, and (5) interacting with nervous system signaling [31].

Nutrient-Specific Modulation of the Microbiome

There is growing interest in targeting gut microbiota through diet and nutritional approaches to promote gut health (management of GI symptoms), mitigate risk factors related to cardiometabolic conditions (CVD, obesity, and diabetes), and treatment of bowel diseases (inflammatory bowel disease). Macronutrients (carbohydrates, proteins, and fats) play a significant role in influencing the gut microbiome. The type of macronutrient (e.g., type of carbohydrate) can further influence the microbiome response including growth, selection of certain species, and synthesis of microbiome metabolites. This section will discuss the effects of macronutrients on the microbiome, with particular attention to relevant clinical conditions.

Carbohydrates

Carbohydrates exist in various forms and influence the gut microbiome through multiple mechanisms. While digestible carbohydrates (e.g., lactose and sialic acid) are quickly processed and used for metabolism, indigestible carbohydrates (e.g., cellulose, pectins, and resistant starch) serve as substrates for microbial fermentation. Diets rich in indigestible fibers are associated with higher abundances of *Prevotella* and *Xylanibacter* species. In particular, increased intake of resistant starch has been linked to greater relative abundance of Bacillota, especially *Ruminococcaceae* [32].

Glycans, complex carbohydrate molecules, are naturally present in foods such as fruits, vegetables, whole grains, and dairy products. Dietary glycans and simple carbohydrates constitute the primary energy sources for gut microbes. When dietary carbohydrate availability is limited, microbial communities may shift toward utilizing host-derived glycans [33].

Proteins

Microbial protein metabolism influences gut microbial composition through two main pathways. In saccharolytic fermentation, amino acids are converted into SCFAs and other bioactive metabolites that generally benefit host health [34]. In contrast, proteolytic pathways generate nitrogenous byproducts such as ammonia, hydrogen sulfide (H_2S), and *p*-cresol, which have been linked to dysbiosis, epithelial barrier dysfunction, and inflammation [35]. In the distal colon, where fermentable carbohydrates are limited, proteolytic activity predominates and produces metabolites that may impair gut and metabolic health. Shifting microbial metabolism toward saccharolytic fermentation could therefore be beneficial in preventing or managing metabolic diseases.

Dietary strategies that promote saccharolytic activity, such as increasing intake of plant-based proteins (e.g., soy) and diverse fibers, may reduce proteolytic fermentation and increase SCFA production, thereby supporting metabolic health in obesity, diabetes, and non-alcoholic fatty liver disease (NAFLD) [36]. Metabolites derived from carbohydrate and protein fermentation play distinct roles in obesity, insulin resistance, diabetes, and NAFLD. SCFAs and intermediates like succinate may help counteract obesity by increasing energy expenditure, enhancing satiety hormone secretion, and improving appetite regulation.

Lipids

Bile acids (BAs) are secreted in response to dietary fat intake and act as conjugated fatty acids that facilitate lipid digestion. Approximately 5% of these conjugated BAs reach the colon where they undergo bacterial metabolism [37]. Dietary fats influence gut microbiota composition by favoring BA-tolerant bacteria capable of producing toxic metabolites such as H_2S, which is also generated during proteolytic protein metabolism. High-fat diets increase BA secretion, promoting the growth of bile-tolerant species that efficiently metabolize conjugated BAs. This shift elevates secondary BAs and toxic metabolite (e.g., H_2S) levels which can damage the intestinal epithelium and contribute to inflammation and disease [38]. While low concentrations of H_2S may have signaling or protective roles, excessive levels are detrimental to gut integrity and immune function.

Beyond BAs, gut bacteria also modify fatty acids by interacting with their double bonds thereby generating metabolites not synthesized by the host. For instance, bacterial metabolism of linoleic acid produces conjugated linoleic acid, a compound with potential effects on host metabolism and health [39].

Micronutrients

Micronutrients can contribute to gut microbiome composition. Vitamin D supplementation can significantly increase gut microbial diversity. This shift is associated with improved gut health and metabolic outcomes. Vitamin D also modulates bacterial genes involved in folate biosynthesis and amino acid metabolism [39].

Phytochemicals

Plant-derived foods contain nutrients that can be utilized when food is consumed. The plants also retain chemicals and nutrients that provide metabolic support for the plant itself. These substances are known as phytochemicals and are discussed in detail in Chap. 7. Humans can obtain benefits from these phytochemicals by way of physiological and metabolic processes, including the gut microbiota.

Phytochemicals modulate the balance and diversity of gut microbiota. Upon consumption, phytochemicals are broken down by gut bacteria into metabolites creating a bidirectional relationship in which the bacteria break down nutrients, then the nutrient metabolites impact the bacteria. These nutrient metabolites are often more active and better absorbed than the original phytochemicals. Further, bacteria of the gut microbiota determine the type and quantity of metabolites produced [40]. Some phytochemicals are broken down by gut bacteria into smaller compounds that may further modulate inflammatory processes, reduce oxidative stress, and improve metabolic health [41].

Dietary Patterns and Food Processing: Impacts on Gut Microbiome Composition and Function

Dietary patterns exert profound and clinically meaningful effects on the gut microbiome and its metabolites which in turn shape host physiology and disease risk (Table 12.1). Western-type diets are energy-dense, high in hyper-palatable foods, and

Table 12.1 Impact of dietary patterns on gut microbiome composition, function, and clinical health

Diet and description	Notable bacterial changes	Functional and metabolite changes	Impact on physiology	Associated conditions	References
Western diet High caloric content and UPFs, artificial additives High in animal protein such as red and processed meats, high-fat dairy, and sugars Low in fiber, fruits, vegetables, whole grains	↑ *Bacteroides* spp. ↑ *Bilophila* spp. ↑ *Alistipes* spp. ↑ *Blautia* spp. ↑ *Ruminococcus* spp. ↑ *Proteobacteria* spp. ↓ *Roseburia* spp. ↓ *Faecalibacterium* spp.	↓ SCFA production ↓ Secondary bile acid production ↑ Endotoxins ↑ TMA, TMAO	↑ Chronic inflammation ↑ Increased oxidative stress ↑ Immune dysregulation ↓ Mucus layer	↑ Obesity ↑ Chronic diseases of lifestyle ↑ Depression ↑ Metabolic disorders	[42, 43]
Mediterranean diet High intake unprocessed, whole-plant foods (fruits, veg, legumes, nuts), whole grains, olive oil Moderate consumption of fish, poultry, dairy, and red wine Low intake of red meat and sweets	↑ *Faecalibacterium* spp. ↑ *Roseburia* spp. ↓ *Collinsella* spp. ↓ *Ruminococcus* spp.	↑ SCFA production and fermentation pathway ↑ Secondary bile acids ↑ Dietary fiber degradation, pectin degradation, mannan degradation pathway	↑ Gut health ↓ Inflammation	↓ CVD ↓ Obesity ↓ Depression	[42–44]
Plant-based eating (vegetarian, vegan, etc.) Enriched in phytochemicals, host-digestible and indigestible carbohydrates	↑ *Prevotella* spp. ↑ *Bifidobacterium* spp. ↑ *Lactobacillus* spp. ↑ *Bacteroides* spp. ↑ *Akkermansia* spp.	↑ Phytochemicals ↑ SCFA production	↑ Neuroprotection and peripheral blood flow ↑ Endothelial, lung and cognitive function ↑ Intestinal barrier integrity ↓ Inflammation and oxidative stress ↓ Pathogenic bacterial growth	↓ CVD ↓ Cancer	[42, 43, 45]

Ketogenic and low-carbohydrate diets Low-carbohydrate, moderate-protein, and high-fat dietary pattern Replicates the metabolic responses seen during fasting, which elevates circulating ketone bodies	↓ *Bifidobacterium* spp. ↓ Actinomycetota ↓ Bacillota ↓ *Bacteroides* spp.	↑ Hydroxybutyrate ketone levels ↓ Intestinal T_H17 cells ↓ SCFA production	↑ Neuronal biogenesis ↓ Neuroinflammation ↓ Mitochondrial dysfunction	↓ Epilepsy ↓ Alzheimer's disease ↓ Obesity ↓ Cancer	[42]
Dietary approaches to stop hypertension (DASH) diet Heart-healthy diet designed to lower blood pressure Emphasizes foods rich in potassium, calcium, and magnesium, including fresh veggies, fruits, whole grains, lean proteins, and low or no fat dairy Reduce foods with sodium, saturated fats, and sweets	↑ *Eubacterium* spp. ↓ Bacillota/ Bacteroidota ratio	↑ Deoxycholic acid (DCA) ↓ TMAO ↓ LPS, LPB	↓ Blood pressure ↓ Gut barrier permeability	↓ CVD ↓ Obesity	[46–48]

UPF ultra-processed food, *SCFA* short-chain fatty acid, *TMA* trimethylamine, *TMAO* trimethylamine N-oxide, *CVD* cardiovascular disease, T_H17 T-helper 17 cells, *LPS* lipopolysaccharide, *LPB* lipopolysaccharide-binding protein are consistently linked to increased inflammation, immune dysregulation, oxidative stress, and disruption of the mucus barrier [49]. This dietary pattern is associated with a relatively high risk of chronic disease. By contrast, healthier dietary approaches such as the Mediterranean diet, plant-based eating patterns, and the Dietary Approaches to Stop Hypertension (DASH) diet (see Chap. 5) generally demonstrate favorable effects on microbial ecology and function. Certain dietary interventions, including ketogenic or low-carbohydrate diets, may also positively influence the microbiome, though their effects can be distinct from other healthful eating patterns.

Other nutrition interventions (e.g., calorie restriction, intermittent fasting) and specific qualities associated with food processing (e.g., fermented foods, ultra-processed foods [UPFs]) also impact the gut microbiome and host physiology. For example, calorie restriction and intermittent fasting have been shown to remodel the microbiome by enhancing microbial diversity, enriching SCFA-producing taxa, and reducing inflammation [50, 51]. Fermented foods (e.g., yogurt, sauerkraut, and kombucha) increase beneficial bacteria such as *Lactobacillus* and *Bifidobacterium* while generating bioactive metabolites [52].

In contrast, UPFs are typically energy-dense, hyper-palatable, and characterized by a high degree of industrial processing and the addition of various additives (see Chap. 4). These foods are consistently associated with adverse microbiome changes, including reduced microbial diversity, an increase in pro-inflammatory or pathogenic taxa, and impaired GI barrier function [49].

Conclusion

Dietary intake and nutrition are highly influential to the structure and function of the gut microbiome, microbiome-associated metabolites, and downstream health factors (see Fig. 12.2). Here we have discussed the biosynthesis of vitamins and fatty acids, bacterial and metabolic characteristics of the diet-microbiome-metabolome axis, how the microbiome utilizes nutrients, and how certain dietary patterns or components can affect the gut microbiota and overall health.

Recent advances in high-throughput multi-omics techniques and integration have allowed researchers to find correlations between nutrition, the gut microbiome, and metabolome. However, more in-depth studies are needed to determine causation using animal models, clinical research trials, and artificial intelligence tools. Limitations in the field that make comparing nutritional-based microbiome studies challenging include the lack of standardized dietary biomarkers, unclear definition of a healthy microbiome, variability of the starting/baseline microbiome of individuals, and differences in study design including how and when stool is collected for microbiome analysis.

Better understanding of the gut microbiota and their metabolites has the potential for therapeutic use from general fecal microbiota transplants (transplanting the full microbiome) to identifying strain-specific bacteria and/or their components for precision medicine. Likewise, modulation of the gut microbiota and metabolites could occur from personalized dietary advice and monitoring.

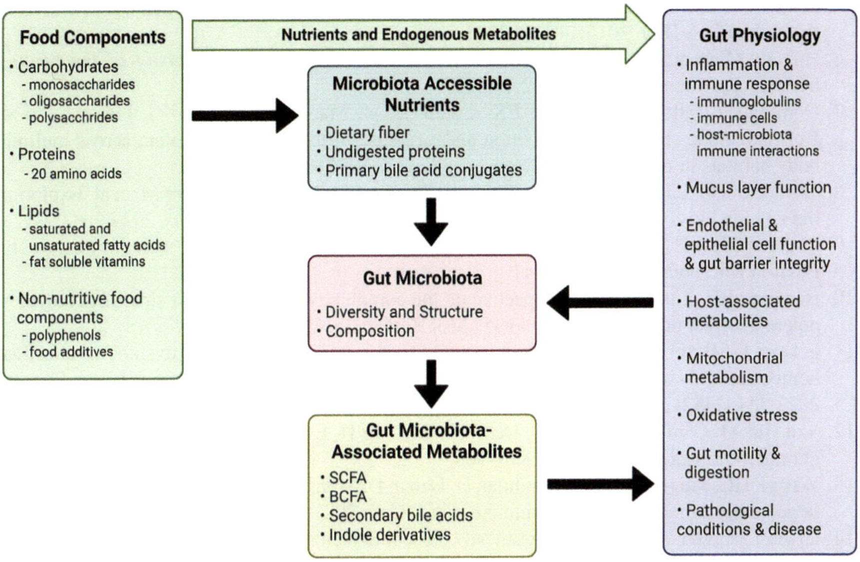

Fig. 12.2 Summary of interactions between food components, the gut microbiome and metabolites, and gut physiology. Food-derived nutrients and non-nutritive components (left panel) provide microbiota-accessible substrates such as dietary fiber, undigested proteins, and primary bile acid conjugates. These substrates shape the diversity, structure, and composition of the gut microbial community (center). In turn, microbial metabolism generates a range of bioactive products, including short-chain fatty acids (SCFAs), branched-chain fatty acids (BCFAs), secondary bile acids, and indole derivatives, which act locally and systemically (bottom). These metabolites and host–microbe interactions influence a variety of physiological processes (right panel), including immune function and inflammation, mucus layer dynamics, gut barrier integrity, mitochondrial and oxidative metabolism, gut motility, and digestion. Dysregulation of these processes can contribute to the development of pathological conditions and chronic disease. Figure (adapted from Zhang [53]).

Disclaimer This research was supported by the Intramural Research Program of the National Institutes of Health (NIH). The contributions of the NIH authors were made as part of their official duties as NIH federal employees, are in compliance with agency policy requirements, and are considered Works of the United States Government. However, the findings and conclusions presented in this paper are those of the authors and do not necessarily reflect the views of the NIH or the U.S. Department of Health and Human Services.

References

1. Oren A. On validly published names, correct names, and changes in the nomenclature of phyla and genera of prokaryotes: a guide for the perplexed. NPJ Biofilms Microbiomes. 2024;10:20.
2. National Center for Biotechnology Information. NCBI Taxonomy to include phylum rank in taxonomic names 2021. https://ncbiinsights.ncbi.nlm.nih.gov/2021/12/10/ncbi-taxonomy-prokaryote-phyla-added. Accessed 17 Oct 2025.
3. National Center for Biotechnology Information. NCBI Taxonomy Browser. 2025.
4. Thursby E, Juge N. Introduction to the human gut microbiota. Biochem J. 2017;474:1823–36.

5. Sender R, Fuchs S, Milo R. Revised estimates for the number of human and bacteria cells in the body. PLoS Biol. 2016;14:e1002533.
6. Human Microbiome Project Consortium. Structure, function and diversity of the healthy human microbiome. Nature. 2012;486:207–14.
7. Dominguez-Bello MG, Costello EK, Contreras M, Magris M, Hidalgo G, Fierer N, et al. Delivery mode shapes the acquisition and structure of the initial microbiota across multiple body habitats in newborns. Proc Natl Acad Sci USA. 2010;107:11971–5.
8. Tarracchini C, Lugli GA, Mancabelli L, van Sinderen D, Turroni F, Ventura M, et al. Exploring the vitamin biosynthesis landscape of the human gut microbiota. mSystems. 2024;9:e0092924.
9. Louis P, Flint HJ. Formation of propionate and butyrate by the human colonic microbiota. Environ Microbiol. 2017;19:29–41.
10. Hamaker BR, Tuncil YE. A perspective on the complexity of dietary fiber structures and their potential effect on the gut microbiota. J Mol Biol. 2014;426:3838–50.
11. Fekete E, Buret AG. The role of mucin O-glycans in microbiota dysbiosis, intestinal homeostasis, and host-pathogen interactions. Am J Physiol Gastrointest Liver Physiol. 2023;324:G452–65.
12. Van Hul M, Cani PD, Petitfils C, De Vos WM, Tilg H, El-Omar EM. What defines a healthy gut microbiome? Gut. 2024;73:1893–908.
13. Wastyk HC, Fragiadakis GK, Perelman D, Dahan D, Merrill BD, Yu FB, et al. Gut-microbiota-targeted diets modulate human immune status. Cell. 2021;184:4137–53.e14.
14. Grace-Farfaglia P, Frazier H, Iversen MD. Essential factors for a healthy microbiome: a scoping review. Int J Environ Res Public Health. 2022;19:8361.
15. Roager HM, Hansen LB, Bahl MI, Frandsen HL, Carvalho V, Gøbel RJ, et al. Colonic transit time is related to bacterial metabolism and mucosal turnover in the gut. Nat Microbiol. 2016;1:16093.
16. Philippot L, Griffiths BS, Langenheder S. Microbial community resilience across ecosystems and multiple disturbances. Microbiol Mol Biol Rev. 2021;85:e00026–0.
17. Fassarella M, Blaak EE, Penders J, Nauta A, Smidt H, Zoetendal EG. Gut microbiome stability and resilience: elucidating the response to perturbations in order to modulate gut health. Gut. 2021;70:595–605.
18. Lozupone CA, Stombaugh JI, Gordon JI, Jansson JK, Knight R. Diversity, stability and resilience of the human gut microbiota. Nature. 2012;489:220–30.
19. Patloka O, Komprda T, Franke G. Review of the relationships between human gut microbiome, diet, and obesity. Nutrients. 2024;16:3996.
20. Culp EJ, Nelson NT, Verdegaal AA, Goodman AL. Microbial transformation of dietary xenobiotics shapes gut microbiome composition. Cell. 2024;187:6327–45.e20.
21. Carmody RN, Turnbaugh PJ. Host-microbial interactions in the metabolism of therapeutic and diet-derived xenobiotics. J Clin Invest. 2014;124:4173–81.
22. Heinken A, Hulshof TO, Nap B, Martinelli F, Basile A, O'Brolchain A, et al. A genome-scale metabolic reconstruction resource of 247,092 diverse human microbes spanning multiple continents, age groups, and body sites. Cell Syst. 2025;16:101196.
23. Luo J, Wang Y. Precision dietary intervention: gut microbiome and meta-metabolome as functional readouts. Phenomics. 2025;5:23–50.
24. Fusco W, Lorenzo MB, Cintoni M, Porcari S, Rinninella E, Kaitsas F, et al. Short-chain fatty-acid-producing bacteria: key components of the human gut microbiota. Nutrients. 2023;15:2211.
25. Oliver A, Chase AB, Weihe C, Orchanian SB, Riedel SF, Hendrickson CL, et al. High-fiber, whole-food dietary intervention alters the human gut microbiome but not fecal short-chain fatty acids. mSystems. 2021;6:e00115–21.
26. Pandey H, Goel P, Srinivasan VM, Tang DWT, Wong SH, Lal D. Gut microbiota in non-alcoholic fatty liver disease: pathophysiology, diagnosis, and therapeutics. World J Hepatol. 2025;17:106849.

27. Yi L, Li Z, Xu H, Shi D, Huang Y, Pan H, et al. Microbiota-based intervention alleviates high-fat diet consequences through host-microbe environment remodeling. Nutrients. 2025;17:1402.
28. Liu TC, Kern JT, Jain U, Sonnek NM, Xiong S, Simpson KF, et al. Western diet induces paneth cell defects through microbiome alterations and farnesoid X receptor and type I interferon activation. Cell Host Microbe. 2021;29:988–1001.e6.
29. Tang WHW. Dysregulated amino acid metabolism in heart failure: role of gut microbiome. Curr Opin Clin Nutr Metab Care. 2023;26:195–200.
30. Boven L, Akkerman R, de Vos P. Sustainable diets with plant-based proteins require considerations for prevention of proteolytic fermentation. Crit Rev Food Sci Nutr. 2025;65:2829–39.
31. Calvanese CM, Villani F, Ercolini D, De Filippis F. Postbiotics versus probiotics: possible new allies for human health. Food Res Int. 2025;217:116869.
32. DeMartino P, Cockburn DW. Resistant starch: impact on the gut microbiome and health. Curr Opin Biotechnol. 2020;61:66–71.
33. Sonnenburg ED, Sonnenburg JL. Starving our microbial self: the deleterious consequences of a diet deficient in microbiota-accessible carbohydrates. Cell Metab. 2014;20:779–86.
34. Diether NE, Willing BP. Microbial fermentation of dietary protein: an important factor in diet¯microbe¯host interaction. Microorganisms. 2019;7:19.
35. Herrera M, Byerley LO. Dietary nitrogen and its role in the gut microbiome and inflammatory bowel disease: a narrative review. Nutrients. 2025;17:2373.
36. Rinninella E, Cintoni M, Raoul P, Lopetuso LR, Scaldaferri F, Pulcini G, et al. Food components and dietary habits: keys for a healthy gut microbiota composition. Nutrients. 2019;11:2393.
37. Ma H, Wang K, Jiang C. Microbiota-derived bile acid metabolic enzymes and their impacts on host health. Cell Insight. 2025;4:100265.
38. Jiang S, Miao Z. High-fat diet induces intestinal mucosal barrier dysfunction in ulcerative colitis: emerging mechanisms and dietary intervention perspective. Am J Transl Res. 2023;15:653–77.
39. Schoeler M, Caesar R. Dietary lipids, gut microbiota and lipid metabolism. Rev Endocr Metab Disord. 2019;20:461–72.
40. Cassidy A, Minihane AM. The role of metabolism [and the microbiome] in defining the clinical efficacy of dietary flavonoids. Am J Clin Nutr. 2017;105:10–22.
41. Wan MLY, Co VA, El-Nezami H. Dietary polyphenol impact on gut health and microbiota. Crit Rev Food Sci Nutr. 2021;61:690–711.
42. Ross FC, Patangia D, Grimaud G, Lavelle A, Dempsey EM, Ross RP, et al. The interplay between diet and the gut microbiome: implications for health and disease. Nat Rev Microbiol. 2024;22:671–86.
43. Randeni N, Bordiga M, Xu B. A comprehensive review of the triangular relationship among diet-gut microbiota-inflammation. Int J Mol Sci. 2024;25:9366.
44. Perrone P, D'Angelo S. Gut microbiota modulation through Mediterranean diet foods: implications for human health. Nutrients. 2025;17:948.
45. Fackelmann G, Manghi P, Carlino N, Heidrich V, Piccinno G, Ricci L, et al. Gut microbiome signatures of vegan, vegetarian and omnivore diets and associated health outcomes across 21,561 individuals. Nat Microbiol. 2025;10:41–52.
46. Baldeon AD, Holthaus TA, Khan NA, Holscher HD. Fecal microbiota and metabolites predict metabolic health features across various dietary patterns in adults. J Nutr. 2025;155:1795–803.
47. Diao Z, Molludi J, Latef Fateh H, Moradi S. Comparison of the low-calorie DASH diet and a low-calorie diet on serum TMAO concentrations and gut microbiota composition of adults with overweight/obesity: a randomized control trial. Int J Food Sci Nutr. 2024;75:207–20.
48. Tilves C, Yeh HC, Maruthur N, Juraschek SP, Miller ER, Appel LJ, et al. A behavioral weight-loss intervention, but not metformin, decreases a marker of gut barrier permeability: results from the SPIRIT randomized trial. Int J Obes. 2022;46:655–60.
49. Maki KA, Sack MN, Hall KD. Ultra-processed foods: increasing the risk of inflammation and immune dysregulation? Nat Rev Immunol. 2024;24:453–4.

50. Shi H, Zhang B, Abo-Hamzy T, Nelson JW, Ambati CSR, Petrosino JF, et al. Restructuring the gut microbiota by intermittent fasting lowers blood pressure. Circ Res. 2021;128:1240–54.
51. Zheng X, Wang S, Jia W. Calorie restriction and its impact on gut microbial composition and global metabolism. Front Med. 2018;12:634–44.
52. Leeuwendaal NK, Stanton C, O'Toole PW, Beresford TP. Fermented foods, health and the gut microbiome. Nutrients. 2022;14:1527.
53. Zhang P. Influence of foods and nutrition on the gut microbiome and implications for intestinal health. Int J Mol Sci. 2022;23:9588.

Diets for Sustainable Food Systems

13

Andrew Berardy and Joan Sabaté

Abstract

- Food systems are the interconnected processes and systems that utilize natural resources to meet societal demands for food, including the life cycle of food production, consumption patterns, and influences on demands.
- Food systems should provide appropriate nutrition for a growing global population while minimizing negative environmental impacts across the supply chain from production through disposal.
- The types of food produced and consumed have impacts on human and planetary health because of the nutrition they provide, the resources they use, and the pollution they emit.
- Diets that emphasize whole, plant-based, and seasonal foods and reduce food waste support improved health and sustainability outcomes.
- Actions to improve sustainability and health include promoting whole-food, plant-centric diets and working to eliminate subsidies of foods that damage human health and the environment.

A. Berardy (✉)
Department of Geography & Earth Sciences, United States Military Academy, West Point, NY, USA
e-mail: andrew.berardy@westpoint.edu

J. Sabaté
Loma Linda University School of Public Health, Loma Linda, CA, USA
e-mail: JSabate@llu.edu

N. J. Temple, T. Wilson (eds.), *Pocket Primer for Nutritional Health*,
https://doi.org/10.1007/978-3-032-25402-3_13

Introduction

Food is a requirement for life, yet it can also threaten longevity of individuals and humanity overall. Modern diets contribute to a plethora of health problems in addition to requiring substantial natural resources to support and emitting significant levels of pollution [1]. Activities related to food present opportunities to improve both human and planetary health through better decisions [2]. Producers, consumers, distributors, policymakers, and other stakeholders all have the potential to make improvements through their decisions regarding food. These actors and their interactions with food contribute to a broader food system.

Food Systems

Food systems are complex, multifaceted socioecological systems with many actors and conflicting interests across a network with interconnections to other systems driving the current reality [3]. At a basic level, the purpose of a food system, Fig. 13.1, is to transform natural resources into food and meet societal demands, but this currently cannot be done without producing waste [1].

Production, processing, packaging, distribution, marketing, purchasing, consumption, and waste of food are all part of the food system, which should provide safe and healthy diets and support human health in an environmentally sustainable and resilient manner [4]. The environmental impacts of food systems come in two primary forms, which are utilization of natural resources and generation of waste, including pollution. Decisions and activities throughout the food system therefore have implications for resource usage, pollution, and health.

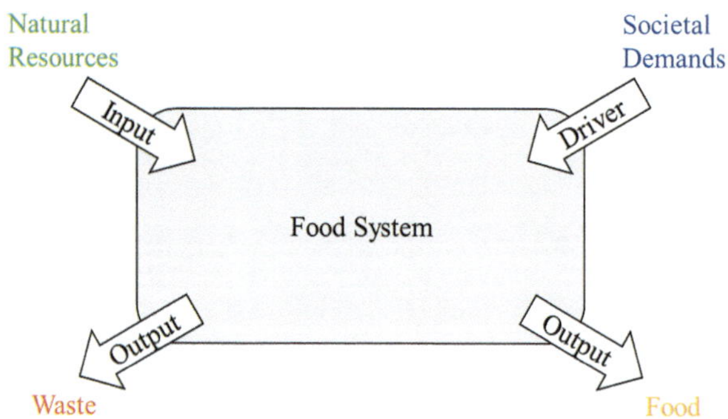

Fig. 13.1 Basic model of a food system. [1]

Environmental Nutrition

Environmental nutrition explores connections between food systems, human health, and the environment, including how the life cycle of food impacts the environment, and how the environment affects food security and nutrition.

Expanding on the basic model of the food system in Fig. 13.1, the environmental nutrition model in Fig. 13.2 outlines the resource inputs necessary to support agriculture and deliver food to consumers, how these are influenced by societal demand, and how these factors combine to determine the outputs of food and waste. The *Environmental Nutrition* textbook covers these concepts in more detail [1].

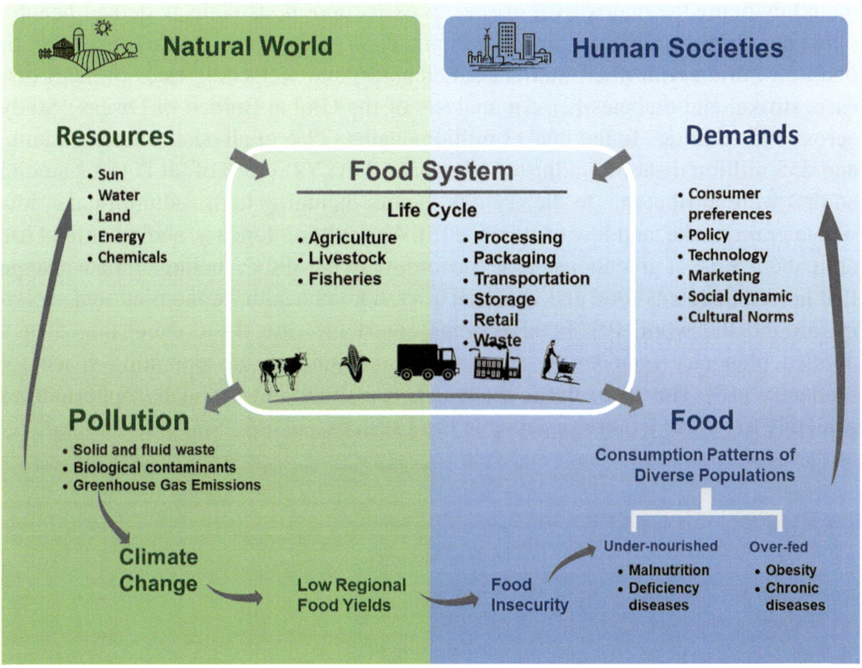

Fig. 13.2 Environmental nutrition model, including interconnected nature of pollution and the food system. [1]

Diet, Health, and the Environment

Modern food systems and food consumption choices have serious negative impacts on the health of humans and the environment. Unhealthy dietary patterns are associated with increases in noncommunicable diseases and mortality [5]. Production and distribution of certain foods cause significantly more environmental damage through resource usage and pollution emissions [6, 7]. As shown in Fig. 13.3 dietary patterns, which shape and are shaped by food systems, influence both planetary and human health, while planetary health influences human health and dietary patterns, forming what has been referred to as a trilemma [8].

The food system uses 70% of the world's freshwater and 40% of its land. Closely related to this, the food system is the largest cause of global environmental changes including being the main driver of species extinction. It also fails to deliver healthy outcomes for the global population which includes 2 billion who are overweight or obese, 2 billion with micronutrient deficiencies, and worsening rates of heart disease, stroke, and diabetes [2]. An analysis of the Global Burden of Disease Study across 195 countries found that 11 million deaths (22% of all deaths among adults) and 255 million disability-adjusted life-years (DALYs) (15% of all DALYs among adults) were attributable to dietary risk factors including high sodium intake, low whole grain intake, and low fruit intake [5]. Agriculture, forestry, and other land use emit about 22% of greenhouse gases according to the IPCC, fueling climate change that in turn threatens food and water security, human health, economies, and societies around the world [9]. Food systems contribute directly to exceeding 5 of 9 defined planetary boundaries necessary to maintain a safe operating space for humanity [10]. However, these challenges also highlight the many opportunities available to pursue a more sustainable food system.

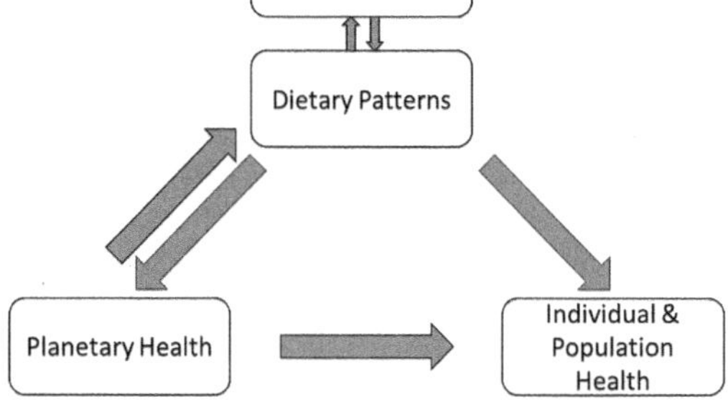

Fig. 13.3 Food systems and dietary patterns are interconnected and influence planetary health and individual population health. Planetary health influences food systems and individual and population health. [1]

Challenges for Sustainable Food Systems

To be considered sustainable, food systems should balance supporting food security, protecting the environment, and providing social benefits [3]. Food security is supported when all people at all times have food availability, accessibility, utilization, and stability [11]. The environment can be protected through optimizing efficiency of production, choosing foods that require fewer resources to produce, and minimizing unnecessary waste [1]. Social benefits of a sustainable food system include employment with adequate income and improving social capital. A sustainable food system must meet societal demands including food security, facilitate positive health outcomes, and minimize resource usage and environmental degradation.

Natural Resources and Environmental Degradation from Food Production

Food production requires use of finite natural resources and also results in changes to landscapes and emissions of pollutants. Researchers have estimated tolerable limits for resource usage and degradation of the environment in order to ensure a safe operating space for humanity. But the food system contributes to exceeding those boundaries in at least five categories, namely climate change, biosphere integrity, land system change, freshwater change, and biogeochemical flows [10]. Agricultural practices contribute to climate change, deforestation, species extinction, water usage, eutrophication, and other resource usage including phosphorus, nitrogen, and fossil fuels [2]. Overall, food systems cause between 11% and 24% of GHG emissions globally, 80–86% of which is from agriculture [4]. Climate change, in turn, is expected to reduce yields and nutrition content of foods, destabilize the food-energy-water nexus, increase reliance on global food trade, and threaten food security [4, 12].

Societal Demands

Globalization, urbanization, and rising per-capita income contribute to the growth of a Westernized diet, which is high in animal-sourced foods, oils, fats, and sweeteners and is associated with negative health and environmental impacts. By the time Earth reaches about 10 billion people in 2050, overall food demand is expected to increase by 50%, and demand for animal-sourced foods is expected to increase by 70% [13].

Some countries are fighting this transition to such an unhealthy and unsustainable dietary pattern or attempting to reverse it [14]. Factors such as policy, marketing, and social dynamics influence consumer preferences, but food choices are also limited by other aspects of food security such as affordability and availability.

Adverse Nutrition and Health Outcomes

Although a balanced diet can promote improved health outcomes, more often diet is a significant driver of noncommunicable diseases. In particular, the Western diet is associated with negative impacts on metabolism, inflammation, cardiovascular health, mental health, and cancer, although these effects can be mitigated by increased physical activity and dietary shifts to increase the proportion of fruits, vegetables, and whole grains [15]. However, dietary guidance and recommendations may be ineffective as demonstrated by the misalignment between Dietary Guidelines for Americans and the diet quality of Americans, with a mean Healthy Eating Index-2015 score of 56.6 out of 100 [4]. Poor food environments, such as food deserts or food swamps, can help drive negative dietary behaviors and associated health outcomes [16].

Sustainability Metrics and Assessment

Determining a sustainable diet is a complex process; it requires a combination of qualitative and quantitative measures. Sustainability's nature as a wicked problem means that an objective measure of sustainability is impossible because subjective judgements are inherent in any potential solution. However, there are ways to quantify differences between foods in their environmental impacts or other dimensions of sustainability.

Life Cycle Assessment

Perhaps the most common quantitative methodology for evaluating the environmental impacts of goods or services, including food, is life cycle assessment (LCA). It is an iterative process that estimates the inputs and outputs associated with the production, distribution, consumption, and disposal of goods, as shown in Fig. 13.4. It determines the anticipated resource usage and emissions associated with the reference flow. The reference flow is a given amount of the product that fulfills the functional unit, which is the basis for estimation and comparison with alternative products and production methods. For example, the functional unit of 1 kg of a food has the same reference flow of 1 kg, but a functional unit of 1 kg of protein from a food has a reference flow of the amount of food necessary to supply that amount of protein [17]. Inputs and outputs for the reference flow are then characterized to estimate the associated environmental impacts.

Types of Environmental Impacts in LCA

Different characterization methodologies quantify different environmental impacts, but most include important categories in resource usage and emissions of pollutants. LCA distinguishes between types of indicators. Midpoint indicators are the direct translation of resource usage and pollution emissions into different types of immediate environmental impacts. Common midpoint indicators include global warming,

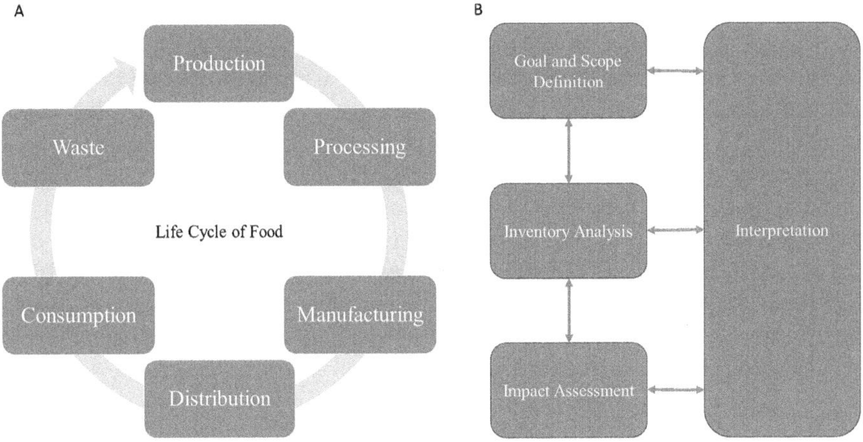

Fig. 13.4 Stages in the life cycle of a product such as food (**a**) and steps in performing a life cycle assessment, showing it as an iterative process (**b**)

land use and transformation, and water consumption. Endpoint indicators aggregate those impacts into broader categories of impact such as human health or ecosystem damage.

Other Methodologies

Although LCA is a robust and widespread methodology, it is insufficient to provide a complete evaluation of sustainability because it has an inherent bias toward efficiency over resilience and only addresses quantifiable impacts [17]. Most assessments of environmental impacts also have limited focus primarily on greenhouse gas emissions from staple crops grown in high-income countries, but the actual impacts depend on where and how food is grown and can vary substantially across many types of impacts [4]. Additional methodologies that can complement an LCA include sustainability assessments, food systems assessments, sustainable materialism, backcasting, and scenario building.

Sustainable Food Systems and Diets

Approaches for Sustainable Food Systems

Possible pathways to pursue a sustainable food system can be classified into three main categories:

1. Production of food
2. Food loss and food waste
3. Consumption patterns

Improvements in production efficiency directly reduce the environmental impact of the current system without requiring changes in consumption patterns. The downside of this approach is that human health impacts will continue to be negative. Reductions in food loss and food waste provide enhanced food security for the population without requiring increases in production, thereby creating a more sustainable food system. This also helps to address human health by increasing nutrient intake in undernourished populations, although it does not address overconsumption. Changes in consumption patterns, and subsequent changes in what is produced, have the greatest potential to achieve a sustainable food system. Through shifting to consumption of lower impact and healthier foods, producers will match this shift, reducing environmental impacts, while at the same time human health will benefit from improved diets.

Foods for Sustainable and Healthy Diets

Sustainable diets must minimize environmental impacts and support human health. Among common characteristics of food, there are four axes with opposing extremes that can guide better decision-making. These are represented in Fig. 13.5. More sustainable diets should trend toward the right side of the spectrum. However, it is important to note that it is not all-or-nothing and there are some potential tradeoffs where increasing one category inherently decreases another.

Animal-Based vs Plant-Based Foods

When animals consume food, they are ingesting only a small portion of the total amount of energy needed to produce that food. The portion of energy thus transferred from one trophic level to another (trophic transfer efficiency) is widely assumed to be about 10%, with empirical evidence showing that it can vary from <1% to 30% [18]. Applying this ecological concept to the food system, it is clear that humans eating animal-based foods is an inefficient use of resources compared

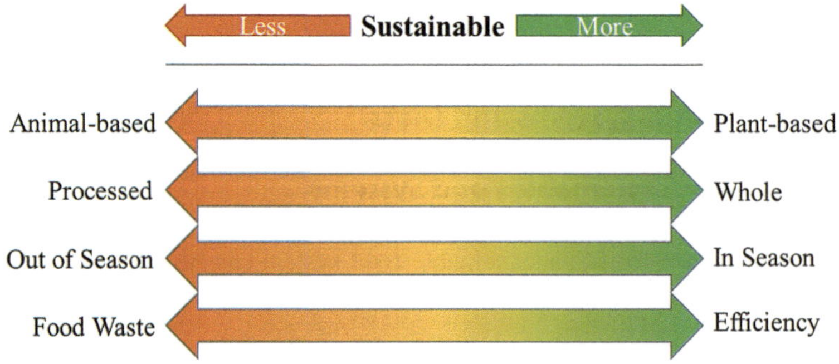

Fig. 13.5 Food-related determinants of sustainable diets

to using those resources to grow food for humans to eat directly. Compared to animal-based foods, plant-based foods are therefore generally more sustainable choices. The superior environmental performance of various plant-centric diets compared to typical or animal-centric diets is supported by a large body of scholarly work, including a systematic review [19]. In fact, even processed plant-based foods have lower environmental impacts than their animal-based counterparts [20, 21].

Processed vs Whole Foods

Processing is done to improve palatability, shelf life, ease of transportation, and safety of foods. However, once a food is available in a safe and edible format, all additional processing unnecessarily increases the environmental impacts associated with that food. Therefore, the more highly processed a food is, the higher its environmental impacts are when compared to a less processed version of that food. Many ultra-processed foods are also eaten for pleasure rather than needed calories, making their environmental impact unnecessary to support a healthy diet [22].

Imported vs Seasonal Foods

Foods that must be delivered further to reach the consumer, especially those which are perishable and need preservation during shipment or faster delivery (e.g., by airplane), have additional environmental impacts compared to those foods that are consumed locally. The concept of food-miles represents the added impact from transportation of food, which is estimated to account for about 19% of total emissions from the global food system [23]. Food miles associated with higher impact foods like meat are a smaller portion of the total than for lower impact foods like vegetables and fruits, making it more likely that importing high-impact foods grown more efficiently elsewhere could be justified [23]. Another important dimension to consider is seasonality, as out-of-season produce typically has additional requirements. For example, use of heated greenhouses substantially increases energy required for production to the point that importing in-season produce from a region where it is produced more efficiently may be environmentally preferable, although this can vary based on specific impacts examined such as water usage [24, 25]. To minimize environmental impacts from production and the supply chain, it makes good sense to prioritize foods that are both in season and locally produced when possible.

Food Waste and Food Loss

The resources used and pollution generated in the production and distribution of food are wasted if that food is not consumed. This results in food loss or food waste. Food loss occurs between the farm and retailer, while food waste occurs between the retailer and consumer [4]. Food waste has larger associated embodied impacts because it occurs further along the supply chain. Both food loss and food waste must be addressed to create a more sustainable food system.

Call to Action

Policymakers should work to support a more sustainable food system while also preserving the food security of their constituents. This goal can be advanced by promotion of healthy and sustainable foods through education, promoting nudges, and even banning excessively harmful foods. To advance efforts for sustainable food systems, policy efforts should simultaneously strive toward just, ethical, and equitable food systems, healthy, adequate, and safe diets for all, economically thriving, robust food value chains, and a clean and healthy planet [26].

Policy must also be supported by science to ensure that recommendations are in line with the reality of the consequences of decisions. Scientists across relevant disciplines including nutrition and environmental science should continue interdisciplinary study of the relationship between food systems and the environment and how to promote transformation into a more sustainable food system in which diets support human and planetary health [4].

Conclusions

Significant challenges to the sustainability of the food system threaten both human and planetary health. Fortunately, simple and actionable recommendations can improve the sustainability of the food system while also promoting personal health. Beneficial changes include reducing or eliminating meat consumption, prioritizing seasonal and whole plant foods, and minimizing food waste. Researchers can support the advancement of sustainable foods by using life cycle assessment to provide a quantitative basis for comparison when there is ambiguity regarding the optimal choice for the environment among foods serving similar functions. Finally, policymakers can shift subsidies away from unhealthy and unsustainable foods in favor of promoting foods that will improve both outcomes instead.

References

1. Springmann M. Can diets be both healthy and sustainable? Solving the dilemma between healthy diets versus sustainable diets. In: Sabate J, editor. Environmental nutrition. San Diego: Elsevier; 2019. p. 197–227.
2. Willett W, Rockström J, Loken B, Springmann M, Lang T, Vermeulen S, et al. Food in the Anthropocene: the EAT–Lancet Commission on healthy diets from sustainable food systems. Lancet. 2019;393:447–92.

3. Eakin H, Connors JP, Wharton C, Bertmann F, Xiong A, Stoltzfus J. Identifying attributes of food system sustainability: emerging themes and consensus. Agric Hum Values. 2017;34:757–73.
4. Fanzo J, Bellows AL, Spiker ML, Thorne-Lyman AL, Bloem MW. The importance of food systems and the environment for nutrition. Am J Clin Nutr. 2021;113:7–16.
5. Afshin A, Sur PJ, Fay KA, Cornaby L, Ferrara G, Salama JS, et al. Health effects of dietary risks in 195 countries, 1990–2017: a systematic analysis for the Global Burden of Disease Study 2017. Lancet. 2019;393:1958–72.
6. Clark M, Springmann M, Rayner M, Scarborough P, Hill J, Tilman D, et al. Estimating the environmental impacts of 57,000 food products. Proc Natl Acad Sci USA. 2022;119:e2120584119.
7. Berardy A, Fresán U, Matos RA, Clarke A, Mejia A, Jaceldo-Siegl K, et al. Environmental impacts of foods in the adventist health study-2 dietary questionnaire. Sustainability (Switzerland). 2020;12:1–14.
8. Tilman D, Socolow R, Foley JA, Hill J, Larson E, Lynd L, et al. Energy. Beneficial biofuels—the food, energy, and environment trilemma. Science. 2009;325:270–1.
9. Calvin K, Dasgupta D, Krinner G, Mukherji A, Thorne PW, Trisos C, et al. IPCC, 2023: climate change 2023: synthesis report. Contribution of Working Groups I, II and III to the Sixth Assessment Report of the Intergovernmental Panel on Climate Change [Core Writing Team, Lee H, Romero J, editors]. Geneva: IPCC; 2023.
10. Richardson K, Steffen W, Lucht W, Bendtsen J, Cornell SE, Donges JF, et al. Earth beyond six of nine planetary boundaries. Sci Adv. 2023;9:eadh2458.
11. Pérez-Escamilla R. Food and nutrition security definitions, constructs, frameworks, measurements, and applications: global lessons. Front Public Health. 2024;12:1340149.
12. Berardy A, Chester MV. Climate change vulnerability in the food, energy, and water nexus: concerns for agricultural production in Arizona and its urban export supply. Environ Res Lett. 2017;12:1–13.
13. Searchinger T, Waite R, Hanson C, Ranganathan J. Creating a sustainable food future: a menu of solutions to feed nearly 10 billion people by 2050-synthesis report. Washington, DC: World Resources Institute; 2018.
14. Azzam A. Is the world converging to a "Western diet"? Public Health Nutr. 2021;24:309–17.
15. Clemente-Suárez VJ, Beltrán-Velasco AI, Redondo-Flórez L, Martín-Rodríguez A, Tornero-Aguilera JF. Global impacts of Western diet and its effects on metabolism and health: a narrative review. Nutrients. 2023;15:2749.
16. Westbury S, Ghosh I, Jones HM, Mensah D, Samuel F, Irache A, et al. The influence of the urban food environment on diet, nutrition and health outcomes in low-income and middle-income countries: a systematic review. BMJ Glob Health. 2021;6:e006358.
17. Berardy A, Johnston CS, Plukis A, Vizcaino M, Wharton C. Integrating protein quality and quantity with environmental impacts in life cycle assessment. Sustainability (Switzerland). 2019;11:2747.
18. Mehner T, Attermeyer K, Brauns M, Brothers S, Hilt S, Scharnweber K, et al. Trophic transfer efficiency in lakes. Ecosystems. 2022;25:1628–52.
19. Hallström E, Carlsson-Kanyama A, Börjesson P. Environmental impact of dietary change: a systematic review. J Clean Prod. 2015;91:1–11.
20. Kustar A, Patino-Echeverri D. A review of environmental life cycle assessments of diets: plant-based solutions are truly sustainable, even in the form of fast foods. Sustainability (Switzerland). 2021;13:9926.
21. Berardy AJ, Rubín-García M, Sabaté J. A scoping review of the environmental impacts and nutrient composition of plant-based milks. Adv Nutr. 2022;13:2559–72.
22. Anastasiou K, Baker P, Hadjikakou M, Hendrie GA, Lawrence M. A conceptual framework for understanding the environmental impacts of ultra-processed foods and implications for sustainable food systems. J Clean Prod. 2022;368:133155.
23. Li M, Jia N, Lenzen M, Malik A, Wei L, Jin Y, et al. Global food-miles account for nearly 20% of total food-systems emissions. Nat Food. 2022;3:445–53.

24. Webb J, Williams AG, Hope E, Evans D, Moorhouse E. Do foods imported into the UK have a greater environmental impact than the same foods produced within the UK? Int J Life Cycle Assess. 2013;18:1325–43.
25. Theurl MC, Haberl H, Erb KH, Lindenthal T. Contrasted greenhouse gas emissions from local versus long-range tomato production. Agron Sustain Dev. 2014;34:593–602.
26. Hebinck A, Zurek M, Achterbosch T, Forkman B, Kuijsten A, Kuiper M, et al. A sustainability compass for policy navigation to sustainable food systems. Glob Food Sec. 2021;29:100546.

Industry Influence: The Food Environment and Nutrition Policy

14

Julia McCarthy

Abstract

- Unhealthy foods and beverages are ubiquitous and unavoidable, shaping social norms, food preferences, and, ultimately, health.
- Concentrated corporate power enables food and beverage manufacturers to shape food environments, including the grocery store, where people purchase the majority of their calories.
- Actions by the food industry in the political arena help to ensure that industry interests hold sway. Such actions include spending on political campaigns, lobbying, and sponsorships; relationships developed through the revolving door; and the publication of self-serving research.
- Recent policy actions, like sugary drink taxes, could help to ensure that, ultimately, public health interests prevail over special interests.

Introduction

In modern, industrialized nations, exposure to unhealthy products is ubiquitous and unavoidable. The food environment undermines best intentions, exposing individuals to unhealthy food and beverages in schools, restaurants, and sports arenas; on sponsor billboards at concerts and community events; and through advertisements on the radio, in print, and on websites. This exposure shapes social norms, determines food preferences, and, ultimately, predicts future health [1].

Federal, state, and local governments are charged with protecting the public from harm. But supporting dietary health is difficult when industry exerts tremendous

J. McCarthy (✉)
New York Health Foundation, New York, NY, USA
e-mail: mccarthy@nyhealthfoundation.org

N. J. Temple, T. Wilson (eds.), *Pocket Primer for Nutritional Health*,
https://doi.org/10.1007/978-3-032-25402-3_14

influence over the places people purchase and consume food, as well as the public institutions responsible for protecting health.

This chapter explores the commercial determinants of health as they relate to the food and beverage industry [2]. In three sections, it examines the strategies and approaches that food and beverage manufacturers use to shape both the food environment and nutrition policy in their favor. The first describes why unhealthy processed foods are abundant in today's food environments. It focuses on one environment, the supermarket, to help illustrate how business practices can undermine public health. The second section explains the various tactics that industry uses to undercut national nutrition policy—how questionably close relationships with regulators, payments to political powerbrokers, and industry-sponsored research stymy development of effective policy. The final section explores policy actions that could help to curb industry power and support healthy eating.

How Industry Practices Shape Food Environments: The Supermarket as a Case Study

In the United States, there are now almost double the number of calories needed for each person each day [3]. Foods that were scarce for most of human history—those high in salt, sugar, and fat—are now bountiful, and that bounty threatens health [4]. U.S. farm subsidies are partially responsible as they favor the production of commodities like corn, used to make high-fructose corn syrup, over "specialty crops" such as broccoli. Commodities are attractive to companies, not only because subsidies make them cheaper, but also because they are more easily processed, theoretically increasing palatability, marketability, and consumption. Processing enables food and beverage manufacturers to increase profits, which is companies' primary goal in a free-market society.

While a free-market society may be good for business, it is not necessarily good for public health. The rise of neoliberal theory following recessions in the 1970s and 1980s led to deregulation, lower corporate taxes, and a weakened public workforce. These actions have contributed to concentrated corporate power which has in turn allowed businesses to have undue influence over food environments [5].

To illustrate this point, consider the grocery store. From both an industry and a public health perspective, supermarkets are a pinnacle of influence. Americans purchase more than 60% of their calories from these stores [6]. Supermarkets, like most food environments, are not nutritionally neutral spaces where you are as likely to find carrots as you are to find candy. One study assessing in-store placement and promotion found that, on average, sugary drinks appear in 25 and other types of unhealthy food in 40 different places across the store [7].

Trade promotion fees are the primary means through which food and beverage manufacturers influence purchasing habits in supermarkets. These companies pay retailers more than $50 billion a year in trade fees to promote their packaged goods [8]. These marketing fees help to explain why healthier foods like fruits and vegetables rarely appear outside of the produce section. Produce companies and farmers cannot afford these fees, and they are not the only ones to lose out: consumers are exposed to fewer healthy options. Trade promotion fees also influence prices. Two-for-one deals, half-off sales, coupons—these are all methods that manufacturers make available to the retailer to ultimately entice customers to buy more. For people who must pay careful attention to food prices, this form of marketing is particularly powerful [9].

Category management is another way manufacturers have been able to tie stores' sales so closely to their own. With category management, the dominant manufacturer in a product category competes for the opportunity to track the performance of products and propose a shelf plan to the retailer. In theory, the category manager makes impartial recommendations not only about where their products should be placed on the shelves but also where their competitors' products are placed, and sometimes how those products are priced. In practice, companies like Coca-Cola are able to decide not only how many slots their traditional sodas will get but also if competitors' healthier products, such as LaCroix, will even appear in the beverage aisle. Category managers are tasked with "growing the category", that is increasing sales. So it is unsurprising that since the practice of category management has taken off, it is the center of the store devoted to shelf-stable goods, not the produce section, that has grown in size as a proportion of the supermarket footprint.

How Industry Influences National Nutrition Policy

Protective policies could disrupt food and beverage manufacturers' practices in the numerous settings where people purchase and consume food. Instead of asking consumers to repeatedly say "no" to unhealthy food, policies could make it easier for everyone to say "yes" to eating healthfully. But the efforts by industry to influence agency officials, politicians, and research can weaken the power of governments to pass and enforce such policies.

Roadblocks to Effective Regulation

One reason why implementing effective nutrition policies in the United States can be difficult is because the responsibility to reduce diet-related diseases is fragmented [10]. Twenty-one agencies oversee approximately 200 different education and clinical services, food access, and regulatory efforts. Of these 21 agencies, the United States Department of Agriculture (USDA) and Health and Human Services (HHS) are the two most relevant. Every 5 years, the USDA, along with HHS, publishes the *Dietary Guidelines for Americans*, forming the basis for all federal nutrition policy and programs. The USDA also regulates and funds many food access and benefits programs, including the Supplemental Nutrition Assistance Program (SNAP). Within HHS, the Food and Drug Administration (FDA) regulates calorie labeling on menus, the Nutrition Facts label and health claims on food packages, and fortification of vitamins and minerals. The Centers for Disease Control and

Prevention (CDC) funds national nonprofits, state governments, and community groups so that they are able to implement strategies for improving community nutrition. And the Federal Trade Commission (FTC) regulates advertising, bringing enforcement actions against companies for deceptive or unfair marketing. The FTC also has subpoena power, meaning it can compel companies to provide information on their business practices.

This fragmentation can reduce the ability of governmental agencies to efficiently and effectively regulate, potentially eroding trust in these institutions. Another mechanism that erodes trust is the "revolving door": industry leaders gain employment in the government agencies that regulate them and vice versa. In theory, the flow of employees between the two sectors can facilitate the flow of knowledge and experience which is potentially useful to both parties. But the "revolving door" can also tip decision-making in favor of industry. Food company executives who join government can stymy policies that could negatively impact the bottom line of their former companies. Conversely, officials entering industry can use their connections to influence regulatory actions.

There are many examples of this practice. In 2017, USDA Secretary Perdue appointed Kailee Tkacz, a former lobbyist for the Corn Refiners Association, as a policy advisor. Though Tkacz had no training in science, public health, or nutrition, White House counsel issued a waiver allowing her to work on the federal *Dietary Guidelines* update, a process she had lobbied on only the year before [11]. Organizations representing food and beverage manufacturers were not shy about leveraging their relationship with her. Records show Tkacz received numerous emails from her former employers. For example, they proposed names for potential members of a federal advisory committee [12]. These emails demonstrate the subtle, often underappreciated, ways that relationships established through the revolving door can influence policymaking. Tkacz currently serves as USDA Chief of Staff, following a brief interim stint as President of the National Oilseed Processors Association.

Paying for Political Power

Another way that industry shapes nutrition policy in its favor is through payments to politically powerful players. Political contributions and lobbyists help open the doors for companies to have access to officials who can influence the writing, enforcement, and retraction of laws and regulations. And industry greatly outspends nonprofits. The following example illustrates this. The Healthy Hunger Free Kids Act is a landmark in child nutrition legislation. In the year that it passed, and the two subsequent years, the nation's largest nutrition advocacy organization spent $70,000 on lobbying—roughly the same amount that industry spent every 13 hours in their lobbying activities [13].

Recognizing that citizens hold great sway over elected officials, food and beverage manufacturers also spend money sponsoring community organizations. Some of these are legitimate while others are front groups. Take, for example, Americans Against Food Taxes (AAFT), the lead group that opposed a national effort to pass a sugary drink tax. On its Facebook page, AAFT claimed to be "a coalition of concerned citizens–responsible individuals, financially strapped families, small and large businesses in communities across the country." But, of the 500 member groups, 73% were affiliated with the food and beverage industry, and only 7% were community organizations. Ninety-three percent of the community organizations for which there were available data were sponsored by industry, and 83% were sponsored by Coca-Cola [14]. As one journalist explained, "AAFT smelled like Astroturf, or corporate lobbyists posing as a grass-roots organization" [15].

Sponsoring community organizations can create pressure for them to participate in front groups; it can also cause them to distance themselves from officials responsible for creating and implementing policy. The experience of New York City Department of Health in 2015 provides a salient example. That year, Coca-Cola, Dr. Pepper, and PepsiCo launched a self-regulatory program, the Balance Calorie Initiative to "help" reduce the number of calories that Americans consume from beverages by 20% by 2025. With the Balance Calorie Initiative, the manufacturers were essentially playing offense as a form of defense, committing to promote lower calorie and smaller portion beverages in pilot neighborhoods like the Bronx [16]. That same year, the Coca-Cola Foundation gave more than $1 million to New York nonprofits, including a $125,000 grant to the Bronx Overall Economic Development Corporation to "promote health, wellness, and physical activity" and a $25,000 grant to a nutrition education group working with Bronx elementary students [17]. Shortly after, Department of Health officials found themselves uninvited from meetings and community events. Longstanding partners explained that it would be "uncomfortable" to have both a representative from the Balance Calorie Initiative and the Department of Health present. As to the question of whether this voluntary industry initiative helped to improve the local food environment, early evaluation from other neighborhoods suggests not [17].

Junk Science in Support of Junk Food

A third industry strategy is to sponsor studies. These studies commonly sow consumer confusion, undercut important policymaking processes, and act as alternative "evidence" in industry-driven litigation. Take, for example, a PepsiCo-sponsored 2021 review of under-consumed food groups and nutrients in the United States, which recommended SNAP policy improvements [18]. The review highlighted oatmeal, popcorn, rice, pasta, and citrus juice as among the most cost-effective sources of under-consumed food groups and nutrients. It concluded that these items "could easily be included (if not already in) in the USDA's Thrifty Food Plan" which serves as the basis for SNAP benefit allotments. Unsurprisingly, PepsiCo produces all highlighted items.

Industry-sponsored studies not only emphasize the positive aspects of their products but can also shift the responsibility for the negative health impacts of the products [19]. For example, decades-worth of research funded by the sugar industry has minimized the link between sugar and heart health [20]. A 2016 literature review examining the relationship between sugary drink consumption, obesity, and diabetes identified 34 studies that found an association, and 26 that did not. Of the studies finding no association, all were industry-sponsored [21].

Countering industry-sponsored studies can consume valuable agency resources. Additional research, communications campaigns, and media may be necessary to debunk distorted science. Creation of the *2020–2025 Dietary Guidelines for Americans* (DGA) process helps to illustrate the threat industry-sponsored science presents to sound policy. In 2020, federal agencies solicited comments for topics to be covered by the *Guidelines*. More than two-thirds of comments submitted were from industry and included "ill-cited and baffling recommendations aimed at skewing the 2020-2025 DGA" [22]. For example, an industry group backed by Coca-Cola cited research by the International Life Sciences Institute (ILSI) stating that low- and no-calorie sweeteners are "safe and effective tools in reducing sugar and overall calories." Founded by a former Coca-Cola executive, ILSI has been criticized for championing business interests that undermine health, such that the World Health Organization (WHO) revoked ILSI's access to its meetings. Mars withdrew its membership, citing ILSI's support for "advocacy-led studies" as the reason [23]. A group responsible for producing and promoting distorted science should not be in a position to influence nutrition policy, but that was the case with the 2020–2025 DGA. The DGA committee is responsible for reviewing current dietary science and reporting the findings. The work of members forms the basis for the DGA and influences national education messages, consumer materials, and nutrition programs. In 2020, more than half of the DGA committee members had ties to ILSI [19].

Finally, industry's manipulation of data matters because it impacts the outcome of court cases. Such was the case in 2015 when San Francisco passed a law that would have required warning labels on sugary drink advertisements, including those on bus stops and billboards. Specifically, advertisements for sugary beverages had to include the following: "WARNING: Drinking beverages with added sugar(s) contributes to obesity, diabetes, and tooth decay."

The American Beverage Association, among other industry actors, contested the law, alleging that it violated their freedom of speech and unjustly targeted sugar-sweetened beverages as a factor in the obesity epidemic [19]. At the district level, the court considered whether the warning was "purely factual and uncontroversial." It concluded that by focusing on a single beverage category, the warning conveyed that these beverages were more likely than other sources of added sugars to harm health. The court relied heavily on industry studies that contradict the established body of evidence. On appeal, the Ninth Circuit decided for industry on different, procedural grounds. Nevertheless, this case demonstrates how industry-sponsored research can undermine government efforts to protect health.

How Policies Can Put People's Health Before Profits

Despite concerted efforts by the food industry to undermine sound nutrition policy, lawmakers continue to push for laws and regulations that improve the food environment. In recent years, national lawmakers have passed policies that have improved transparency, by, for example, requiring added sugars to be disclosed on the back of products. Others have gone further, removing trans fat from the food supply and updating the nutrition standards for meals served in schools.

Federal policy change can be difficult given the level of consensus needed. Nevertheless, federal policymakers continue to take steps to improve the food environment. For example, after two decades and multiple requests from advocacy groups, in late 2021 the FTC launched an investigation of industry practices in supermarkets, requiring many companies to share their pricing, marketing, promotions, and brand selection strategies with the agency [24]. Findings from this investigation informed a report that found that during COVID, these large players "accelerated and distorted the negative effects associated with supply chain disruptions" [25]. And in 2024, the agency took legal action to block two of the nation's largest supermarkets, noting the potential harm to consumers; nine attorneys general (AGs) joined the suit [26].

At the state level, AGs may also play an important role in policy enforcement, bringing needed attention to public health issues [27]. For example, in 2009, an AG investigated the Smart Choices Program. This is a self-regulatory program run by industry which labeled store products like Frosted Flakes as healthy. The investigation prompted the FDA to initiate its own investigation and ultimately led to industry ending the program.

A number of promising retail policies are gaining momentum at the local level. Sugary drink excise taxes are one such example. Although levied on the manufacturer, the tax is passed on to the consumer at the point of purchase, usually the supermarket. These taxes discourage consumption, raise local government revenue, and encourage manufacturers to reduce the sugar content of their products. In 2014, Berkeley, California, became the first U.S. jurisdiction to pass such a tax. An evaluation 3 years later showed sugary drink consumption in low-income neighborhoods had fallen by more than 52% [28]. Since Berkeley's passing, seven additional U.S. jurisdictions have implemented sugary drink taxes.

Conclusions

Food and beverage manufacturers produce many of the salty, sweet, and tempting foods that clutter food environments. The supermarket is just one example of an environment where unchecked business practices can undermine health. In the political arena, fragmentation and revolving door practices weaken regulatory agencies' ability to check that power. At the same time, campaign donations and sponsorships coupled with self-serving research conspire to advance the interests of the food industry.

As former World Health Organization Director-General Chan has noted, “Efforts to prevent non-communicable diseases go against the business interests of powerful economic operators.” [29]. But promising policies could help to ensure that going forward, public health interests prevail over special interests. Evaluation of such policies—real research, not distorted science—will help determine what combination best supports healthy eating. And, with the public increasingly interested in healthy options, support for such policies is likely to grow.

References

1. Kraak V, Gootman J, McGinnis JM. Food marketing to children and youth: threat or opportunity? Institute of Medicine. 2006. https://nap.nationalacademies.org/catalog/11514/food-marketing-to-children-and-youth-threat-or-opportunity. Accessed 5 Nov 2025.
2. Kickbusch I, Allen L, Franz C. The commercial determinants of health. Lancet Glob Health. 2016;4:e895–6. https://www.thelancet.com/journals/langlo/article/PIIS2214-109X(16)30217-0/fulltext
3. Roser M, Ritchie H, Rosado P. Total daily supply of calories per person, 1961 to 2022. Our World in Data. December 2023. https://ourworldindata.org/food-supply. Accessed 5 Nov 2025.
4. Cohen DA. A big fat crisis. New York: Nation Books; 2014.
5. Lencucha R, Thow AM. How neoliberalism is shaping the supply of unhealthy commodities and what this means for NCD prevention. Int J Health Policy Manage. 2019;8:514–20.
6. Mancino L, Guthrie J. U.S. Department of Agriculture Economic Research Center. Supermarkets, schools, and social gatherings: where Supplemental Nutrition Assistance Program and other U.S. households acquire their foods correlates with nutritional quality. 2018.
7. Cohen DA, Bogart L, Castro G, Rossi AD, Williamson S, Han B. Beverage marketing in retail outlets and the balance calories initiative. Prev Med. 2018;115:1–7.
8. The Goldman Sachs Group Inc. U.S. consumer packaged goods and retail: trade budgets at a tipping point. 3 November 2015.
9. Darmon N, Drewnowski A. Contribution of food prices and diet cost to socioeconomic disparities in diet quality and health: a systematic review and analysis. Nutr Rev. 2015;73:643–60.
10. U.S. Government Accountability Office. GAO-21-593: federal strategy needed to coordinate diet-related efforts. August 2021. https://www.gao.gov/products/gao-21-593. Accessed 5 Nov 2025.
11. Union of Concerned Scientists. Betrayal at the USDA: how the Trump administration is sidelining science and favoring industry over farmers and the public. April 2018. https://www.ucsusa.org/sites/default/files/attach/2018/04/betrayal-at-the-usda-report-ucs-2018.pdf. Accessed 5 Nov 2025.
12. Peterson L. Project on government accountability. the snack food and corn syrup lobbyist shaping Trump's Dietary Guidelines for Americans. 23 August 2018. https://www.pogo.org/investigations/the-snack-food-and-corn-syrup-lobbyist-shaping-trumps-dietary-guidelines-for-americans. Accessed 5 Nov 2025.
13. Wilson D, Roberts J. Special report: how Washington went soft on childhood obesity. Reuters. 27 April 2012. https://www.reuters.com/article/world/special-report-how-washington-went-soft-on-childhood-obesity-idUSBRE83Q0EE/. Accessed 5 Nov 2025.
14. Yanamadala S, Bragg MA, Roberto CA, Brownell KD. Food industry front groups and conflicts of interest: the case of Americans Against Food Taxes. Pub Health Nutr. 2012;15:1331–2.
15. Cohen R. An anti-tax argument that's hard to swallow. The New York Times 21 September 2009. https://ethicist.blogs.nytimes.com/2009/09/21/an-anti-tax-argument-thats-hard-to-swallow/. Accessed 5 Nov 2025.

16. Coca-Cola. New York City joins Alliance for a Healthier Generation and America Beverage Association Balance Calories Initiative. 27 May 2015. https://www.einnews.com/pr_news/267648707/new-york-city-joins-alliance-for-a-healthier-generation-and-america-beverage-association-balance-calories-initiative. Accessed 5 Nov 2025.
17. The Coca-Cola Foundation. Grants paid in 2015 by organization. 2015. https://www.yumpu.com/en/document/read/55266179/the-coca-cola-foundation-grants-paid-in-2015-by-organization. Accessed 5 Nov 2025.
18. Brauchla M, Fulgoni VL. Cost-effective options for increasing consumption of under-consumed food groups and nutrients in the USA. Pub Health Nutr. 2021;25:710–6.
19. Roache SA, Platkin C, Gostin LO, Kaplan C. Big food and soda versus public health: industry litigation against local government regulations to promote healthier diets. Fordham Urb Law J. 2018;45:1051–89.
20. Kearns CE, Schmidt LA, Glantz SA. Sugar industry and coronary heart disease research: a historical analysis of internal industry documents. J Am Med Assoc Internal Med. 2016;176:1–2.
21. Schillinger D, Tran J, Mangurian C, Kearns C. Do sugar-sweetened beverages cause obesity and diabetes? Industry and the manufacture of scientific controversy. Annals Internal Med. 2016;165:895–7.
22. Corporate Accountability. Dietary guidelines for corporate America. 16 June 2020. https://www.corporateaccountability.org/resources/dietary-guidelines-corporate-america/2020-06-16-dgac-media-brief_corporate-accountability_final/. Accessed 5 Nov 2025.
23. Jacobs A. A shadowy industry group shapes food policy around the world. The New York Times. 16 September 2019. https://www.nytimes.com/2019/09/16/health/ilsi-food-policy-india-brazil-china.html. Accessed 5 Nov 2025.
24. U.S. Federal Trade Commission. FTC launches inquiry into supply chain disruptions. 29 November 2021. https://www.ftc.gov/news-events/news/press-releases/2021/11/ftc-launches-inquiry-supply-chain-disruptions. Accessed 5 Nov 2025.
25. U.S. Federal Trade Commission. FTC releases report on grocery supply chain disruptions. 21 March 2024. https://www.ftc.gov/news-events/news/press-releases/2024/03/ftc-releases-report-grocery-supply-chain-disruptions#:~:text=The%20report%20revealed%20that%20large%20market%20participants,as%20the%20impacts%20on%20consumers%20and%20businesses. Accessed 5 Nov 2025.
26. U.S. Federal Trade Commission. FTC challenges Kroger's acquisition of Albertsons. 26 February 2024. https://www.ftc.gov/news-events/news/press-releases/2024/02/ftc-challenges-krogers-acquisition-albertsons. Accessed 5 Nov 2025.
27. Pomeranz JL, Brownell KD. Advancing public health obesity policy through state attorneys general. Am J Pub Health. 2011;101:425–31.
28. Lee MM, Falbe J, Schillinger D, Basu S, McCulloch CE, Madsen KA. Sugar-sweetened beverage consumption 3 years after the Berkeley, California sugar sweetened beverage tax. Am J Pub Health. 2019;109:637–9.
29. World Health Organization. WHO Director-General addresses health promotion conference. 10 June 2013. https://www.who.int/director-general/speeches/detail/who-director-general-addresses-health-promotion-conference

An Overview of Key Advances in Nutrition: More Than the Sum of the Parts

15

Norman J. Temple and Karen Davison

Abstract

- This chapter provides a summary of some of the key advances achieved in nutrition science in recent decades. Most of the topics covered were discussed in more detail in earlier chapters.
- Several new topics are covered including dietary recommendations, back-of-package food labels, the potential hazards of toxic chemicals in food, and false and misleading claims.
- The information presented in this chapter shows how health may be enhanced and diet-related diseases prevented. There is clearly a great opportunity to achieve a major improvement in the well-being of the population by the application of nutrition science.
- This chapter presents a summary of the key lessons from this book and the top priorities for action in the broad area of nutrition.

N. J. Temple (✉)
Centre for Science, Athabasca University, Athabasca, AB, Canada
e-mail: normant@athabascau.ca

K. Davison
Institute for Life Course and Aging, University of Toronto & The Centre of Clinical Excellence, Toronto, ON, Canada

Centre for Science, Athabasca University, Athabasca, AB, Canada
e-mail: karend@athabascau.ca

N. J. Temple, T. Wilson (eds.), *Pocket Primer for Nutritional Health*,
https://doi.org/10.1007/978-3-032-25402-3_15

Introduction

In recent years, we have seen major leaps forward in nutrition science. This has been seen in all areas, from bench science to population health. As a result, a much greater understanding of the relationship between diet, the causes of chronic diseases of lifestyle (CDL), and how to maintain good health has been realized. These discoveries offer the realistic promise of major improvements in many areas of health across the population and greatly reducing the burden of CDL.

This chapter provides a summary of some of the key advances. Most of the topics covered were discussed in more detail in earlier chapters. In addition, a few new topics are covered including back-of-package food labels, the potential hazards of toxic chemicals in food, and false and misleading information in nutrition.

Dietary Patterns

Chapter 5 explored healthier alternatives to the Western diet. Currently, it appears the Mediterranean diet (MD) has the strongest supporting evidence and consensus among scientific and professional communities related to the prevention of CDL. Prospective cohort studies, randomized controlled trials, systematic reviews, and meta-analyses have revealed that consumption of the MD beneficially affects health outcomes related to CVD and all-cause mortality. Many countries have adapted versions of the MD to align with regional cultural food preferences and integrate principles of environmental sustainability.

Other healthier alternatives to the Western Diet to highlight include the Dietary Approaches to Stop Hypertension (DASH), the Portfolio Diet (PD), other regional-based guidelines such as the Nordic and Asian diets, and variations of vegetarian diets. Of these, the DASH has clearly shown positive effects on blood pressure and cardiometabolic outcomes. Similarly, the PD improves lipid and blood glucose profiles and blood pressure as well as reducing the risk of all-cause mortality. The MIND (Mediterranean-DASH Intervention for Neurodegenerative Delay) diet leverages aspects of the MD and DASH and appears to have various cognitive-related benefits.

A major goal is to shift the dietary pattern consumed by the majority of the population away from the Western diet. Towards that end vegetarian diets and the Planetary Health Diet (PHD) may be especially beneficial as they not only improve population health but also help achieve the goals of environmental sustainability. Carefully planned vegetarian diets show promise in improving body composition, metabolic health, gut microbiome composition, and inflammation, mainly among populations of high- and middle-income countries. Vegan-oriented eating patterns and the PHD, which recommends dairy and animal protein intake to not exceed 9% of total energy intake, have been positively associated with healthier body composition and cardiometabolic indicators plus environmental indicators such as the carbon footprint and water usage.

All of the diets referred to in this chapter share similar key features which include consuming generous amounts of vegetables, fruit, whole grains, and plant protein sources such as nuts, legumes, and seeds. These foods are major sources of phytochemicals. As described in Chap. 7 an impressive weight of evidence has accumulated showing that these substances are associated with a reduced risk of a wide variety of CDL. Fatty fish are rich in n-3 fatty acids and can also make a valuable addition to the diet.

Ultra-processed foods (UPF) are the diametric opposite of healthy foods. These foods are a major part of the Western diet. Many cohort studies have reported that persons who have a relatively high intake of UPF are at an increased risk of a wide range of poor health outcomes (Chap. 4). But it would be a mistake to conclude that there is a simple cause-and-effect relationship between intake of UPF and risk of various diseases. The problem is that UPF are poorly defined. Many relatively healthy foods meet the definition of UPF. One example is breakfast cereals that contain processed whole grains plus various additives. Conversely, various unhealthy foods are not classed as UPF (e.g., red meat that has been minimally processed). Based on the totality of the current evidence, UPF should be viewed as being a crude indicator of unhealthy foods. However, in one area, namely obesity, there is strong evidence that implicates UPF in disease risk. The supporting evidence was discussed in section "Ultra-processed foods and obesity" of Chap. 4.

Dietary Recommendations, Recommended Nutrient Intakes, and Food Guides

Recommendations for Nutrient Intake

The set of recommendations for nutrient intake in the USA is known as the Recommended Dietary Allowances (RDA). First published in 1943 it has been revised multiple times. The Dietary Reference Intakes (DRI) is a development of the RDA. It gives reference values of estimated nutrient requirements that can be used across the lifespan [1, 2]. The DRI include four tables including estimated nutrient requirements (the RDA and Adequate Intakes) and an estimate of safe maximal intake (Tolerable Upper Intake Levels). These tables are used in the USA and Canada and are intended to assist clinicians, dietitians, and the general public in planning and assessing the dietary intake of healthy individuals.

Values of RDA are given for 14 vitamins, 15 minerals, energy, carbohydrates, protein, dietary fiber, water, and n-3 and n-6 polyunsaturated fatty acids. Tables are broken down by age and sex. Specific recommendations are given for women who are pregnant or lactating.

Like all expert pronouncements in the field of nutrition there is a lack of consensus over some aspects of the contents of the DRI. Nutritional science has evolved and some guidelines, such as vitamin D and fat, would benefit from review and updating. In addition, for some nutrients, such as chromium, there is debate about their essentiality [3].

Dietary Guidelines

Different countries publish sets of dietary guidelines with the goal of improving the diets eaten by the population. The primary goal is to reduce the burden of CDL. The American version is known as the *Dietary for Guidelines Americans* (DGA). It is produced jointly by the U.S. Department of Agriculture (USDA) and the U.S. Department of Health and Human Services (HHS) [4]. A new version is published every 5 years. The current version covers the period 2020–2025. It provides dietary advice for people of all ages and all stages of the lifespan. The DGA is adaptable to different ethnic groups.

The large majority of the DGA comprises advice that can be readily understood by the general public. But the DGA also includes quantitative recommendations intended for health professionals. These set upper limits on the intake of saturated fatty acids, sugar, salt, and alcohol.

Food Guides

Countries around the world publish food guides. These are a type of dietary advice for the population in the form of a simple pictorial representation of the recommended diet [5, 6]. For many years, the food guide used in the USA was shaped like a pyramid. Earlier versions were known as the *Food Guide Pyramid* but the name was later changed to *MyPyramid.* In 2011, the USDA replaced this design with a simple pictorial design called *MyPlate* [7]. This elegantly simple food guide is in the form of a plate with food sectors (Fig. 15.1). The area of the plate given to each food group indicates what proportion of the diet should come from that food group, much like the old *Food Guide Pyramid. MyPlate* places little emphasis on how many servings should be eaten from each food group which is a radical departure

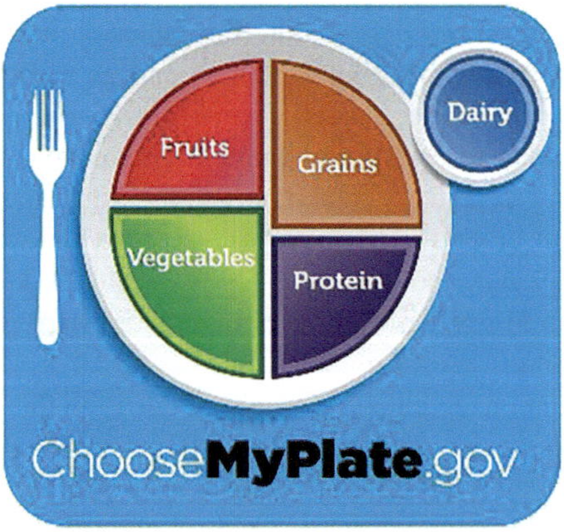

Fig. 15.1 MyPlate USDA design [7]. (Reprinted from U.S. Department of Agriculture)

from the design of the *Food Guide Pyramid* and *MyPyramid*. However, recommendations for serving sizes are included on the *MyPlate* website.

Clear trends are seen in the design of food guides used in different countries. First, increasing numbers of countries, including Canada and the UK, have adopted a dinner plate design. Second, these food guides now provide little or no advice regarding how many servings should be consumed from each food group. Third, food guides have much increased the proportion of the diet that should come from fruit, vegetables, and whole grains while de-emphasizing meat.

Food Labels

Food labels are very much a work in progress. They come as two main types, namely front-of-package (FOP) food labels and back-of-package (BOP) food labels. Both types are intended to help and encourage consumers to select healthier foods.

Front-of-Package Food Labels

The different types of FOP labels were described in Chap. 10. While many research studies have been carried out, it has not been established which labels are most successful in terms of achieving a positive impact on the behavior of consumers so that they select healthier foods.

The most promising findings about FOP initiatives have come from graded summary labels. Nutri-Score is the most well-known design of this type and is widely used in Europe. It assigns one of five grades, from the healthiest (A) to the unhealthiest (E), each accompanied by a different color. This grading is based on the overall healthiness of the food and considers many ingredients in the food such as fruit, vegetables, fiber, sugar, sodium, and vitamins.

Warning labels are a type of interpretive single nutrient-specific label. Typical examples are "High in Salt" and "High in Sugar". This label design has been adopted by many countries in the Americas.

FOP labels hold much promise for helping consumers select a healthier diet. For that reason, these labels are potentially a valuable tool for improving food and nutrition literacy and for health promotion. However, there is still much uncertainty regarding which design is most effective and the extent to which FOP labels have a positive impact on population diets when used in real-world situations such as supermarkets. While most FOP labels impact consumer behavior positively, the best evidence suggests that their impact is relatively small in real purchase situations and on overall diet quality.

Back-of-Package Food Labels

The BOP food label used in the USA and Canada are known as the Nutrition Facts Label. They are very similar but with some differences. The label lists the nutritionally important nutrients or other components found in a food. The current design used in the USA was introduced in 2020. A typical example of it is shown in Fig. 15.2. The label is required only for food sold in packages, such as cans or cardboard boxes, but not for other foods, such as fresh meat and fish.

The label focuses on nutrients that are associated with certain chronic diseases or with nutrient deficiencies. The label must contain the following information:

- List of ingredients arranged in descending order by weight (main ingredient first).
- Serving size (using a standardized serving size), plus the number of servings per container. For packages that contain more than one serving, the label states the nutrition information per serving as well as per package.
- Amount per serving of the following: total calories, fat, total fat, saturated fat, trans fat, cholesterol, sodium, total carbohydrate, dietary fiber, total sugar, pro-

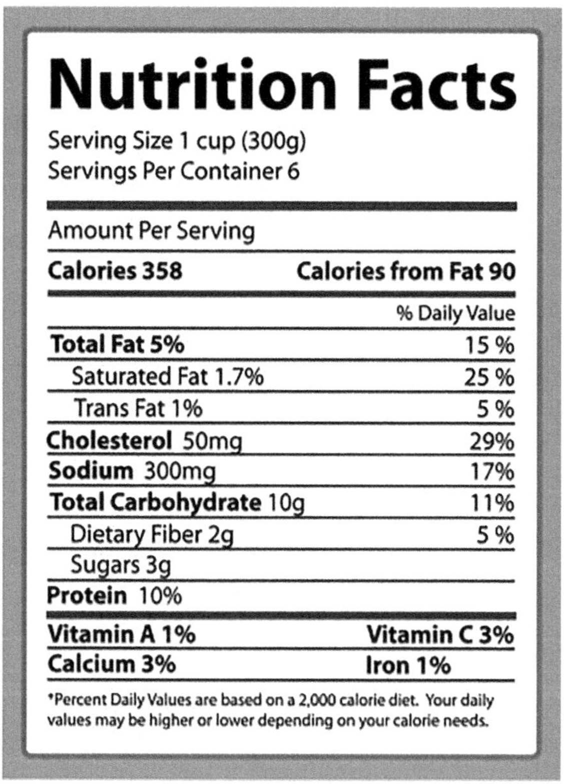

Fig. 15.2 Example of the Nutrition Facts Label as used in the USA

tein, vitamin D, potassium, calcium, and iron. These quantities are also listed for the whole package for foods that are typically consumed in one sitting. However, if the food has a negligible amount of a particular food component, then it may be omitted from the label.
- The sugars listed on the label include naturally occurring sugars (such as those in fruit and milk) as well as those added to a food or drink.
- If the product is making a claim for a particular nutrient, information for that nutrient must be included.

Diets for Sustainable Food Systems

A development in the field of nutrition science in recent years has been the realization that food production has a major impact on multiple aspects of the environment. In particular, food production often involves the production of vast quantities of greenhouse gases and is therefore an important contributor to climate change. Food production is also the largest cause of global environmental changes including being the main driver of species extinction and deforestation, as well as using enormous amounts of water. This subject is examined in Chap. 13.

There is now a growing recognition that radical change is needed in how food is produced. This subject is referred to as food sustainability. Foods of animal origin, most notably meat, have by far the most impact on the environment. For that reason, the diets eaten around the world need to shift to ones dominated by plant foods while the amount of commonly consumed meats need to be much reduced.

Sustainability requires a broadly based strategy that includes placing greater emphasis on seasonal foods and reducing food waste. Another goal is the elimination of subsidies for the production of foods that damage the environment.

Adopting the goals of food sustainability can and should be done in conjunction with moving towards healthier diets. Indeed, there are already steps in that direction. Chapter 5 described the Planetary Health Diet. That diet is designed to be both sustainable and healthy. This approach needs to be extended to other areas of dietary advice including food guides and food labels [8]. For example, the Nutri-Score food label could be reformulated so that it indicates both how healthy and sustainable a given food item is. This strategy could potentially help achieve both human and planetary health.

Health Promotion

The Limited Success of Health Promotion

As documented throughout this book, great progress has been made in understanding how the diet commonly eaten in the USA and Western countries should be changed in order to achieve major progress in improving population health and preventing CDL. Over the past 40 years, a great many health promotion campaigns have been carried out. They have attempted to persuade people to follow a healthy lifestyle, especially in the areas of diet, exercise, and weight management. People have been targeted via the mass media, in the community (including in schools), at the worksite, in the physician's office, or via social media. Unfortunately, these campaigns have only achieved a limited degree of success. Of particular importance, risk of CVD (including CHD) is likely to be reduced by about 5–15%. But there is little positive impact on the majority of people at risk. Thus, it can be assumed that efforts to encourage people to lead a healthier lifestyle will not achieve a major impact on the proportion of people succumbing to CDL.

The same conclusion is reached when the enormous efforts to persuade the general population to adopt a healthier diet are examined. These include such educational tools as food guides, food labels, and messages delivered through mass media channels. Progress has been painfully slow. This was documented in Chap. 9 (section "Is the population adopting a healthier lifestyle?"). This is epitomized by the obesity epidemic. This emerged in the USA around 1978. The fundamental cause is undoubtedly related to an unhealthy lifestyle. Yet there is little or no evidence of progress in stopping the epidemic, let alone reversing it.

Nutrition Policy by Governments

Chapter 9 also surveyed nutrition policy by governments. This covered such topics as lowering the salt content of food, placing restrictions on the advertising of unhealthy foods, and the use of taxes and subsides in order to make healthy foods more affordable relative to less healthy foods. The chapter presents the case that (in comparison with the health promotion strategy described above) a strategy based on government policy is likely to achieve much more success in encouraging the population to adopt a healthier lifestyle including a healthier diet. Another important advantage of this strategy is that it is cost-effective.

A Strategic Plan

There is an urgent need for a comprehensive action plan [9] aimed at improving nutrition-related outcomes. This includes a combination of education, advice, and encouragement, including health promotion, as well as action policies by governments. The goal of this plan is to foster an environment that makes healthy choices in diet and other aspects of lifestyle the easy and affordable choices. A brief summary is as follows:

1. Provide subsidies that encourage consumption of healthier foods combined with adding taxes on unhealthy foods.
2. Enact stricter regulation of adverts for unhealthy foods. Of most importance, adverts for foods of low diet quality should be banned when the target audience is children.

3. Improve the design of food labels so that they are more user-friendly and encourage healthy food selection behaviors (see Chap. 10).
4. Set strict limits on the content of food ingredients and additives known to negatively impact health if consumed in excess.
5. The government should, where feasible, exert pressure on key food environments, such as schools and other publicly-funded institutions, so that they provide healthy food. This policy could serve as a guiding principle for government programs that provide food assistance to people on low incomes.
6. Health promotion campaigns that have demonstrated effectiveness should be expanded.

This plan has the potential to achieve a major advance in population health. The World Cancer Research Fund International made similar proposals with a plan known as NOURISHING [10].

Dietary Supplements

The possible benefits of dietary supplements have been much debated for decades. The interpretation of the literature presented in Chap. 6 makes the case that solid supporting evidence exists for only a small minority of the supplements presently being marketed.

There is a compelling case for the benefit of taking a vitamin D supplement. This is especially the case for population groups who are most likely to have low blood levels of the vitamin. These include persons with dark skin and those with limited exposure to the sun such as frail older people and people who live in the northern states of the USA or in Canada. A commonly recommended dose is around 1000 IU (25 μg) per day.

A large body of evidence demonstrates that fatty fish is protective against CVD. The fats that deliver this benefit are long-chain n–3 polyunsaturated fatty acids. It follows, therefore, that people should be advised to eat at least one or two servings of fatty fish per week. Examples of fatty fish include salmon, herring, mackerel, sardines, and pilchards. But many people do not consume fatty fish or only eat small amounts. For these people, there is a strong case for dietary supplements of fish oil. The case is especially strong for those who have CVD or are at high risk of the disease.

Probiotics are supplements that contain particular bacteria in a concentrated form. Evidence from controlled trials has demonstrated that particular probiotics are beneficial for colon function. This may be of value in both prevention and therapy of diverse range of health conditions. The strongest evidence has been reported for their use in the prevention of urinary tract infections in women, respiratory tract infections, and antibiotic-associated diarrhea. Probiotics have also been reported to enhance the immune response. While the use probiotics as dietary supplement holds much promise, it is premature to recommend them for the general population. One reason for this is that the formulation of probiotics is highly variable and much is still unknown about the individual and synergistic effects of particular strains.

Multivitamins refer to pills that contain a broad selection of vitamins and minerals and that are typically taken once a day. They are the most commonly taken dietary supplement. Many millions of Americans take this supplement and no doubt believe that they help safeguard health. But there is little evidence that the large majority of users gain any benefit to their health. It may, however, be a different story with particular groups. In particular, people who may benefit from taking multivitamins are those at risk of malnutrition such as people who habitually consume a low-calorie diet which is often the case with elderly people and those with anorexia, drug addiction, or advanced cancer.

The rapid rate at which nutrition science is advancing makes it highly likely that important discoveries of valuable new supplements will be made in the coming years. As documented in Chap. 7, the broad field of phytochemicals is a likely place where such discoveries will be made.

The Need for Providing Nutrition Education for Medical Students and Trained Doctors

This book has documented the enormous weight of evidence that demonstrates the central importance of nutrition in the prevention and therapy of a wide variety of diseases and health disorders. This leads to the obvious conclusion that physicians need a solid knowledge of nutrition in order to successfully carry out their work. Alas, in this area progress has been underwhelming.

It is well established that physicians typically have major weaknesses in their knowledge of nutrition [11]. This problem reflects the serious lack of nutrition education in medical schools. A review was carried out of nutrition education in medical schools across the USA [12]. The findings showed serious deficits in the teaching of nutrition. Valuable insights into this problem were gained from a systematic review carried out on medical students, mostly in the USA, Europe, and Australasia [13]. The findings revealed that the students had a poor knowledge of nutrition as well as limited confidence in their ability to implement nutrition care for their patients.

These problems have been well known for more than 40 years. For example, a study in 1977 documented this problem among American physicians [14]. Likewise, a recent review pointed out that the need for nutrition education in American medical schools was proposed in 1985 in a report from the National Academies yet in 2025 there was little evidence of real progress [15].

The Dangers to Health Posed by Food Corporations

There is a long history of food corporations giving the highest priority to maximizing profits regardless of the damage done to the health of the population. The same picture is seen with corporations coming from a variety of industries. The tobacco industry illustrates this perfectly. Starting in the 1950s evidence steadily accumulated revealing that smoking is a major cause of cancer and other diseases. The tobacco industry then spent decades telling anyone who would listen that the rock solid scientific evidence was wrong. The motive was to block, as far as possible, any actions, such as restrictions on marketing or increased taxes on tobacco products, that might reduce sales and profits. The pharmaceutical industry has had numerous scandals over the past half century where unsafe drugs have been marketed while legitimate safety concerns have been glossed over. In several such cases, consumer profits are the primary goal while the people prescribed the drug have suffered real harm. The greatest scandal concerns opioids. Starting around 1991, there was an enormous increase in the marketing of these drugs for pain relief. Physicians were told that they pose only a small risk of addiction. This was patently untrue. Massive overprescribing appears to have been a major factor in setting off an enormous epidemic of opioid addiction and death. This epidemic is especially widespread in the USA, where well over 800,000 people have died as a result. But many other countries have also been affected.

The massive use of fossil fuels is the major cause of climate change. This poses enormous threats to the livelihoods of future generations. It is therefore a matter of great urgency that major cuts are made to the use of fossil fuels. But this poses a threat to the massive profits made by the fossil fuel industry. Major parts of the industry have shown little hesitation in placing their profits above the health of the planet and its population. Key parts of their game plan include distorting the scientific evidence and lobbying governments so that only policies favorable to the fossil fuel industry are implemented.

The practices of food corporations have much in common with the corporations discussed above. On countless occasions, food corporations have prioritized the production and marketing of unhealthy foods, such as ultra-processed foods, at the expense of healthy food choices. This was described in Chap. 14. The evidence presented in that chapter demonstrates that the actions of the food industry succeed in thwarting the hard work carried out by health professionals in their efforts to encourage the population to consume a healthier diet.

The Suspected Danger of Toxic Chemicals in Food

For decades, a great many people have expressed alarm over the potential hazards related to industrial chemicals that enter the environment, many of which end up to the food we eat. In December 2025, a report was released authored by an international team of experts [16]. The report focused on four families of industrial (synthetic) chemicals that are widely present in food. These are

- Phthalates and bisphenols. These are used for many reasons such as plastic additives and as food packaging.
- Pesticides. These are used in enormous quantities in agriculture in order to eliminate weeds and insects. Additionally, many crops are treated with pesticides after harvest to maintain freshness.

- PFAS (polyfluoroalkyl substances), also known as "forever chemicals". They have received much publicity in recent years. They are used in food contact materials such as greaseproof paper, popcorn tubs, and ice-cream cartons. They can remain in the environment for decades where they can enter food via air, soil, and water.

These four families of industrial chemicals have been linked to a variety of harmful effects in humans including endocrine disruption, cancer, birth defects, cognitive impairment, and obesity. They also pose multiple risks to the environment.

These substances are subject to much weaker degrees of regulation than is the case with pharmaceuticals. It is a case of safe until proven dangerous rather than the reverse which is the case with new drugs.

The estimated cost of these chemicals is $1.4 to $2.2 trillion per year, which equates to 2–3% of global gross domestic product (GDP). These figures are considered conservative as they exclude many possible sources of damage from these chemicals, such as loss of biodiversity.

Pseudoscience: The Dangers of False and Misleading Claims in Nutrition

False and misleading claims are a widespread problem across many areas of the medical sciences. This problem has a long history. For example, in Victorian times, it was commonly believed that masturbation leads to blindness and insanity. In recent years millions of parents have been persuaded that some types of vaccination pose a significant risk to children. The resulting decrease in the proportion of children who have been vaccinated has led to many cases of measles and some deaths. This problem appears to have become more widespread during 2025. The Covid-19 pandemic led to the appearance of vast amounts of fake information across the internet.

In the 1970s, low blood glucose was often cited as the underlying cause of such problems as feeling irritable and lacking in energy. This misleading claim went out of fashion only to be replaced by newer nutrition-related fads such as gluten intolerance, an overload of toxins, and a yeast infection (Candida). The problem of fake science is especially pervasive in nutrition. A major part of the marketing of dietary supplements is based on false and misleading claims [17].

The scope of the problem of false and misleading statements is enormous and is continuously evolving. The Internet serves as an efficient vehicle by which false information can quickly spread around the world. This section presents some illustrative examples of the problem.

Blood Types and Health

In 1991, James D'Adamo published a book with the title "*The Blood Type Diet: Your Personalized Diet and Exercise Program*". The theme of this book is that people should select their diet, as well as their exercise program, based on their ABO blood group. Over the following years, several other authors published books making similar claims such as that a person's blood group is an effective means to both prevent and treat an assortment of health problems including cancer, heart disease, diabetes, arthritis, and overweight. There is no real evidence to support the claims made in these books [18].

The Case of Dr Oz

Dr Mehmet Oz was for many years a highly accomplished heart surgeon at Columbia University, New York. He has had a TV show since 2009 that has been watched by millions of people across North America. He dispenses advice on many topics in the general area of health. Researchers from the University of Alberta in Edmonton, Canada, made a careful analysis of the accuracy of his claims [19]. They estimated that 39% of his advice was in the area of diet. The researchers were able to find evidence in support of 46% of the recommendations while 15% were contradicted by the evidence. That left 39% of the recommendations where no supporting evidence could be found. In other words, at least half of the recommendations made by Dr Oz lacked supporting scientific evidence.

One of his claims landed him in hot water. Dr Oz was called before Congress to testify at a Senate hearing about deceptive advertising for over-the-counter diet supplements after he sang the praises of green coffee bean extract as a "miracle" weight loss pill [20]. Sen. Claire McCaskill, who chairs the Senate's Consumer Protection panel, blasted him for making such claims on his show when "you know it's not true".

Bogus Weight-Loss Treatments

Millions of people in the USA and around the world are desperate for effective treatments that will deliver weight loss. This is an area where huge amounts of highly misleading information are being given. A person who enters a health food store and asks for advice on weight loss will probably receive a recommendation to take one or more supplements. But the advice usually has a serious lack of credible supporting evidence. The problem is also very widespread in the print media. One of the magazines displayed at the checkout in supermarkets across North America is *Woman's World*. Most weeks its front cover has a "lose a pound per day" diet. Vast numbers of diet books have been published in recent decades. The numbers have been expanding at the same rate as American waistlines. The problem of books that disseminate grossly inaccurate information goes far beyond weight loss. Thousands of books on diverse topics related to nutrition have been published but a great many of them are worse than useless.

A Brief Summary

When we make an overview of the current state of nutrition science and practice, we see overwhelming evidence that the application of our present knowledge has the potential to deliver major advances in population health.

The rivers of Montana serve as an analogy with the current situation. One river flows west to the Pacific Ocean, a second goes north through Canada to Hudson Bay and thence to the Atlantic Ocean, and a third joins the Missouri, then the Mississippi, and continues to the Gulf of Mexico. These rivers resemble the world of nutrition and health: many streams flow into major rivers of ideas, action, and direction, but these rivers can flow in opposite directions and interact in complex ways with the total landscape of nutritional health. Over recent decades, several new streams have merged with the rivers.

Until the 1970s and 1980s, the relationship between diet and disease was viewed mainly in terms of the quantities of nutrients in the diet, particularly vitamins, minerals, and fats. But since then paradigm shift has taken place. The component parts of this shift are described in the chapters of this book. In order to properly understand the relationship between diet and disease, it is necessary to integrate all the many complexities of the human diet including the following:

- We now have a far clearer understanding of the relationship between various parts of the diet and risk of disease. Major examples include the protective action of marine fats (long-chain n–3 polyunsaturated fatty acids), vitamin D, and dietary fiber, the harmful effects of sugar, salt, and *trans* fatty acids, and the minor role of the total amount of fat.
- The role of phytochemicals (Chap. 7). An abundance of evidence demonstrates that these substances play a major role in protection against disease.
- The microbiome (Chap. 12). The microorganisms in our bodies, most particularly in the colon, have a major impact on body functioning and on the etiology of many diseases.

Nutrition scientists have traditionally subscribed to the viewpoint that if we can fully understand the role of the above-mentioned substances as well as all the nutrients, and, in addition, the myriad factors that affect metabolism, we can then fully explain the relationship between diet and disease. Moreover, this understanding will enable us to design the healthiest diet. But such a viewpoint is deeply flawed. The reasons for this bring us to the concept of food synergy which was examined in Chap. 8. The central tenet of food synergy is that the relationship between diet and disease cannot be explained in terms of the individual actions of the enormous number of different substances present in food. Rather, diet-related disease is caused by the combined action of these substances, probably acting synergistically. To properly understand the mechanisms involved is a challenge of mind-boggling complexity that will take many decades to achieve. For that reason, the most productive strategy for explaining the relationship between diet and disease and identifying the healthiest diet is to focus on foods and dietary patterns rather than single substances.

But at the same time we recognize the role of single substances when there is solid evidence that they have distinct actions in the body and are clearly linked to risk of particular health conditions. Examples of this include vitamin D, salt, and *trans* fatty acids. In each case, we need to increase or decrease intake as appropriate in order to protect health. But these examples are the exceptions.

Based on this summary of the evidence dietary advice can be stated in very simple terms as follows:

The diet should be based on a healthy dietary pattern such as the Mediterranean diet. But at the same time people should eat fatty fish, take supplements of vitamin D (if there is inadequate exposure to sunshine), and limit intake of sugar and salt.

This dietary advice must be seen within a broader picture. The following areas are of especial importance:

- Nutrition science has little value unless it leads to an improvement in the diet eaten by the general population. For that reason action policies by governments are a high priority. In addition, there should be more funding and support for health promotion so that the population receives more education and encouragement in the area of healthy eating.
- Protection of the environment is another priority. Accordingly, sustainability must be a key component of dietary advice and policy.
- Attempts by food corporations to block or water down efforts to reduce the sale of unhealthy foods must be vigorously resisted.
- Continued research is needed with the following being areas of particular importance: nutrition and genetic interactions; the impact of food production on the environment and how best to meet the goals of sustainability; the details of the functioning of the human gut microbiome and the design of the most effective probiotics; and the search for new and effective dietary supplements.

References

1. Dietary Reference Intakes. Applications in dietary assessment. Washington, DC: National Academies Press; 2000.
2. Institute of Medicine; Otten JO, Hellwig JP, Meyers LD, editors. Dietary reference intakes: the essential guide to nutrient requirements. Washington, DC: The National Academies Press; 2006.
3. Chen J, Kan M, Ratnasekera P, Deol LK, Thakkar V, Davison KM. Blood chromium levels and their association with cardiovascular diseases, diabetes, and depression: National Health and Nutrition Examination Survey (NHANES) 2015–2016. Nutrients. 2022;14:2687.
4. U.S. Department of Agriculture and U.S. Department of Health and Human Services. Dietary guidelines for Americans, 2020–2025, 9th ed. 2020. DietaryGuidelines.gov. Accessed 5 Jan 2026.
5. Montagnese C, Santarpia L, Iavarone F, et al. North and South American countries food-based dietary guidelines: a comparison. Nutrition. 2017;42:51–63.
6. Montagnese C, Santarpia L, Buonifacio M, et al. European food-based dietary guidelines: a comparison and update. Nutrition. 2015;31:908–15.

7. U.S. Department of Agriculture (USDA). MyPlate. 2011. http://www.choosemyplate.gov/index.html. Accessed 5 Jan 2026.
8. Tiboni-Oschilewski O, Abarca M, Santa Rosa Pierre F, Rosi A, Biasini B, Menozzi D, et al. Strengths and weaknesses of food eco-labeling: a review. Front Nutr. 2024;11:1381135.
9. Temple NJ. Strategic nutrition: a vision for the twenty-first century. Public Health Nutr. 2016;19:164–75.
10. World Cancer Research Fund International. 2025. NOURISHING policy Framework | World Cancer Research Fund. Accessed 31 Dec 2025.
11. Temple NJ. Survey of nutrition knowledge of Canadian physicians. J Am Coll Nutr. 1999;18:26–9.
12. Bassin SR, Al-Nimr RI, Allen K, Ogrinc G. The state of nutrition in medical education in the United States. Nutr Rev. 2020;78:764–80.
13. Crowley J, Ball L, Hiddink GJ. Nutrition in medical education: a systematic review. Lancet Planet Health. 2019;3:e379–89.
14. Krause TO, Fox HM. Nutritional knowledge and attitudes of physicians. J Am Diet Assoc. 1977;70:607–9.
15. Albin JL, Thomas OW, Marvasti FF, Reilly JM. There and back again: a forty-year perspective on physician nutrition education. Adv Nutr. 2024;15:100230.
16. Systemiq. Invisible ingredients: tackling toxic chemicals in the food system. Systemiq-Invisible_Ingredients-Tackling_toxic_chemicals_in_the_food_system-EN. 2025. Accessed 28 Dec 2025.
17. Temple NJ. Dietary supplements and health. One part science, nine parts hype. In: Temple NJ, Wilson T, Jacobs DR, Bray GA, editors. Nutritional health: strategies for disease prevention. 4th ed. New York: Humana Press; 2023. p. 389–400.
18. Cusack L, De Buck E, Compernolle V, Vandekerckhove P. Blood type diets lack supporting evidence: a systematic review. Am J Clin Nutr. 2013;98:99–104.
19. Korownyk C, Kolber MR, McCormack J, et, al. Televised medical talk shows—what they recommend and the evidence to support their recommendations: a prospective observational study. BMJ. 2014;349:g7346.
20. Firger J. Dr. Oz defends weight-loss advice at Senate hearing on diet scams. CBS News, June 17, 2015. www.cbsnews.com/news/dr-oz-defends-weight-loss-advice-at-senate-hearing-on-diet-scams. Accessed 20 December 2025.

Appendices

Appendix A: Sources of Reliable Information on Nutrition

Books

Sizer F, Whitney E. Nutrition: Concepts & Controversies, 16th ed. Cengage Learning, 2022.
Whitney E, Rolfes S. Understanding Nutrition, 16th ed. Cengage Learning, 2025.
The above two books are general textbooks that cover all areas of nutrition. They are written for undergraduate university students.
Gropper S, Smith J, Carr T. Advanced Nutrition and Human Metabolism, 8th ed. Cengage Learning, 2021.
This book covers many topics in nutrition with a focus on metabolic aspects.
Katz D, et al. Nutrition in Clinical Practice, 4th ed. LWW, 2022.
Clinical nutrition written for physicians.
Temple NJ, Wilson T, Jacobs DR, Jr, Bray GA, eds. Nutritional Health: Strategies for Disease Prevention, 4th ed. Springer Nature, New York, 2023.
This book covers many areas of nutrition. The book is intended for researchers, physicians, dietitians, and others who wish to study nutrition in depth.
Wilson T, Temple NJ, Bray GA, eds. Nutrition Guide for Physicians and Related Healthcare Professionals, 3rd ed. Humana (Springer), New York, 2022.
This book covers more topics in nutrition but in less depth than the book *Nutritional Health*. The book is intended for physicians, dietitians, and other health professionals.

Internet Websites

Cancer

National Cancer Institute
This provides extensive information on all aspects of cancer including the role of nutrition.
Website: https://www.cancer.gov

N. J. Temple, T. Wilson (eds.), *Pocket Primer for Nutritional Health*,
https://doi.org/10.1007/978-3-032-25402-3

World Cancer Research Fund International
This website covers the same topics as the previous website.
Website: Homepage | World Cancer Research Fund

Cardiovascular and Related Diseases

American Heart Association
A resource on diverse areas of cardiovascular disease.
Website: https://www.heart.org

National Heart, Lung, and Blood Institute
Provides much valuable information on diseases of the heart and respiratory system and related subjects.
Website: https://www.nhlbi.nih.gov

Composition of Foods and Diets

FoodData Central
This website operated by the US Department of Agriculture (USDA) provides a detailed analysis of a wide variety of foods.
Website: USDA FoodData Central

Nutrition Value
Much like the previous website, this website provides a detailed analysis of a wide variety of foods. In addition, it allows individuals to analyze their diet and keep track of their diet over time.
Website: Nutritional Values for Common Foods and Products

General Information

Academy of Nutrition and Dietetics
This website is another source of reliable information across many areas of health and medicine. It has a strong focus on nutrition.
Website: https://www.eatright.org

Mayo Clinic
This is operated by the Mayo Clinic and provides much information on health and disease, including diet and supplements.
Website: https://www.mayoclinic.com

MedlinePlus
This website provides extensive information on many aspects of health and medicine. It is operated by the National Library of Medicine which is part of the National Institutes of Health.
Website: https://medlineplus.gov

MEDLINE and PubMed

MEDLINE is the National Library of Medicine's bibliographic database and contains more than 40 million references to journal articles in thousands of scholarly journals in the life sciences, with a concentration in biomedical sciences. MEDLINE content is searchable via PubMed.

Website: Single Citation Matcher - PubMed

MyHealthfinder

A source of health information on many topics. The website is run by the US Department of Health and Human Services. When checked in May 2026, it was still delivering scientifically accurate information on vaccinations.

Website: MyHealthfinder | odphp.health.gov

Health Fraud

Quackwatch

This organization and its website provide reliable information on a wide range of health frauds.

Website: https://www.quackwatch.org

Other Areas of Health

American Academy of Pediatrics

Information on all aspects of pediatrics including nutrition.

Website: https://www.aap.org

American Diabetes Association

Extensive information on all aspects of diabetes.

Website: https://www.diabetes.org

National Institute on Aging

Information for issues related to aging.

Website: https://www.nia.nih.gov

National Institute of Diabetes and Digestive and Kidney Diseases

Information on diabetes and diseases of the digestive tract, kidney, liver, blood, and urinary tract. Other topics covered include nutrition and weight control.

Website: https://www.niddk.nih.gov

Appendix B: Glossary of Terms

Alpha-linolenic acid (ALA)
An n-3 PUFA found in some plant oils.

Case-control studies
A direct comparison is made between healthy subjects and people who already have the disease of interest. By comparing the exposure of the two groups, the researchers can estimate the extent to which the diet variable (or other lifestyle variable) is associated with the risk of the disease.

Cohort studies (prospective or longitudinal studies)
These are a type of study where subjects are recruited who are free of the disease of interest. After a period of follow-up, the data are analyzed to determine the association between dietary and other lifestyle variables and risk of disease. This type of study is suggestive of a causal association as the exposure and the outcome occurred in a temporal sequence. This is a distinct advantage of cohort studies over case-control studies.

Confounding
This indicates a correlation of the exposure and the outcome with other variables. Such correlation may mask true associations between the diet variable and the outcome or produce false associations. Confounding is of great importance in epidemiological studies as lifestyle factors tend to cluster together.

Cross-sectional studies
Subjects are compare for exposure to the diet variable of interest and the presence of the outcome of interest. With this design, the findings present a snapshot in time. Cross-sectional studies are often used to look at body parameters that increase by increments, such as BMI and blood pressure.

DASH diet (Dietary Approaches to Stop Hypertension)
The diet was originally developed with the primary goal of lowering blood pressure.

EAT-Lancet Commission
This diet was developed in 2019 and is designed to be both healthy and sustainable. It is now known as the Planetary Health Diet.

Epidemiology
The study of the incidence, distribution, control, and prevention of disease.

Flexitarian diet
Type of vegetarian diet characterized by eating plant-based foods, varying amounts of fish and dairy, and lower quantities of meat.

Food synergy
This concept argues that many associations between diet and risk of disease are best understood in terms of the overall effects of foods and dietary patterns, not merely as a collection of individual nutrients and other bioactive substances.

Genome-based personalized nutrition
This integrates genetic, phenotypic, and comprehensive nutrition assessment data to provide precise dietary guidance to help optimize health status.
Genomic medicine. This integrates individual genomic information as part of one's health care.

Guideline Daily Amounts label
Type of front-of-package food label. The label states the amount of sugar, fat, saturated fat, salt, and energy per serving.

Guiding Stars label
Type of front-of-package food label. This is a summary label where the health value of each food is indicated by the presence of from zero to three stars.
Lacto-ovo diet
Type of vegetarian diet that includes dairy products and eggs but excludes meat, poultry, and fish.

Marine fats
This refers to types of fat that are present in fish, especially fatty fish. This fat is predominately long-chain n-3 polyunsaturated fatty acids. The two main fatty acids are eicosapentaenoic acid (EPA) and docosahexaenoic acid (DHA).

Mechanistic research
In this research strategy, researchers attempt to understand the details of body physiology and biochemistry, such as intermediary metabolism. In the field of nutrition, researchers attempt to discover how the various chemicals in food are involved in health or disease.

Mediterranean diet
Diet based on foods traditionally eaten in the countries that border the Mediterranean.

Microbiome
This refers to this community of microorganisms, especially bacteria, along with the collective genomes and gene products of its members.

MIND diet (Mediterranean-Dash Intervention for Neurodegenerative Delay)
A healthy eating plan that integrates the Mediterranean and DASH diets with the goal of reducing the risk of cognitive impairments and dementia.

Monounsaturated fatty acids
Fatty acids with one double bond.

Multiple Traffic Lights label
Type of front-of-package food label. The label states the amount of sugar, fat, saturated fat, salt, and energy per serving. Each part of the label is color coded to indicate if the amounts are high, medium, or low.

NHANES (National Health and Nutrition Examination Survey)
Large ongoing survey that measures health and nutritional status of the population of the United States.

Nordic Diet
Diet designed to be healthy and based on foods traditionally eaten in Nordic countries. It has several variations such as the New Nordic Diet.

NOVA System
Classification system where foods are classified based on the extent to which the food has been processed and the purpose of the processing. One of the food groups is ultra-processed foods (UPF).

Nutrigenetics
This focuses on the effects of inter-individual differences of genetic variants on responses to nutrients and other bioactive food components in relation to disease.

Nutrigenomics
This encompasses genome-based patterns such as DNA methylation, epigenetics, and metabolic regulation influenced by nutritional uptake.

Nutri-Score label
Type of front-of-package food label. This is a summary label where each food is placed in one of five groups from most to least healthy.

Pescatarian diet
Type of vegetarian diet that includes fish and shellfish but excludes meat including poultry.

Phytochemicals
Diverse groups of natural bioactive compounds produced in plants.

Planetary Health Diet
A diet designed to be both healthy and sustainable. It was originally developed in 2019 as the EAT-Lancet Commission.

Polyunsaturated fatty acids (PUFA)
Fatty acids with two or more double bonds.

n-3 (omega-3) PUFA
Type of PUFA. Major sources include fatty fish and some types of vegetable oil.

n-6 (omega-6) PUFA
Type of PUFA. Many vegetable oils are rich in these fats.

Population studies (ecological studies)
Typically, two dozen or more different countries are compared. Data are collected from each country on food intake and exposure to possible risk factors and these are compared with disease rates.

Probiotics
Preparations intended for human consumption that contain particular bacteria in a concentrated form.

Randomized controlled trials (RCTs)
The subjects are randomized into at least two groups: a control group (i.e., untreated, usual care, placebo, or standard treatment) and one or more intervention groups.

Refined grains
Grains that have been processed. As a result their content of micronutrients and fiber is depleted.

Saturated fatty acids (SFA)
Fatty acids with no double bonds.

Sustainable food system
This refers to a food system that supports food security, protects the environment, and provides social benefits.

Systematic reviews and meta-analyses
In a systematic review, the literature is reviewed using search engines according to strict criteria. Relevant information is extracted from each paper that meets the criteria. The findings from these papers are then summarized. A meta-analysis takes this process one step further. The reviewers make pooled risk estimates. Compared with single studies this research strategy generates results that gain power by increasing sample size.

Trans-fatty acids
These are a type of polyunsaturated fatty acid (PUFA). They are formed from PUFA during hydrogenation. This process is often used by food manufacturers to make liquid oils more solid. These fats have a harmful effect on blood lipids. Strong evidence indicates that they increase the risk of CHD.

Ultra-processed foods (UPF)
These are foods that are made from mixtures of ingredients that are the product of industrial processes. UPF contain products extracted from actual foods combined with various additives.

Vegan diet
A strict vegetarian diet that excludes all animal-derived foods.

Warning label
Type of front-of-package food label. The label warns consumers that the food has a high content of unhealthy components such as sugar and salt.

Whole grains
Grains that have been minimally processed. These grains have a relatively high content of micronutrients and fiber.

Index

A

Academy of Nutrition and Dietetics, 125
Action policies, in school, 98–99
Adipokines, 20
Adiposity-based chronic disease (ABCD), 21
Adverse nutrition, 150
Alcohol, CHD/CVD, 31, 32
Alpha-linolenic acid (ALA), 29
American Association of Clinical Endocrinology, 21
American Beverage Association, 162
American Council on Exercise, 125
American Nutrition Association, 125
Americans Against Food Taxes (AAFT), 161
Amino acids, diet-microbiome-metabolite axis, 135
Animal-based foods, 152
  vs. plant-based foods, 153
Anthocyanins, 77
Attention, 112
Attenuation, 5
Attorneys general (AGs), 163

B

Back-of-package food labels, nutrition, 172, 173
Balance Calorie Initiative, 161
Bile acids (BAs)
  diet-microbiome-metabolite axis, 133, 135
  microbiome, 136, 137
Bisphenols, 177
Blood, types and health, 178–179
Body mass index (BMI), 16, 17
Body Roundness Index (BRI), 16
Bogus weight-loss treatments, 179
Bronx Overall Economic Development Corporation, 161

C

Calcium, 66
Canadian Health Check, 111
Cancer, carotenoids, 76
Carbohydrates
  CHD and
    intake, 30
    refined grains, 30
    sugar, 30
    whole grains, 30
  microbiome, 136
Cardiovascular disease (CVD), 26
Carotenoids, 73, 76
  cancer, 76
  cognitive function, 76
  eye diseases, 76
  metabolic-associated diseases, 76
Case-control studies, nutrition research, 5, 6
Category management, 159
Cause-and-effect, 7
Centers for Disease Control and Prevention (CDC), 16, 159–160
Central adiposity, 16
Chinese Healthy Eating Index (CHEI), 54
Chlorogenic acid, 78
Choices label, 111
Chronic diseases of lifestyle (CDL), 47, 94, 118
Chronic relapsing disease process, obesity, 20, 21
Coca-Cola, 161
Coffee, and CHD/CVD, 31, 32
Cognitive function, 76
Cohort studies
  nutrition research, 3–5
  randomized controlled trials *vs.*, 8, 9
Commercial determinants of health, 158
Communities, campaigns in, 94

N. J. Temple, T. Wilson (eds.), *Pocket Primer for Nutritional Health*,
https://doi.org/10.1007/978-3-032-25402-3

Computer-mediated health promotion, 95
Confounding, 5
Consumer behavior, 106
  and FOP food labels, 111–113
Coronary heart disease (CHD), 25, 26, 66
  alcohol, tea, coffee and, 31, 32
  carbohydrates and
    intake, 30
    refined grains, 30
    sugar, 30
    whole grains, 30
  dietary fat and
    fat content of diet, question of, 26
    fish, n–3 polyunsaturated fatty acids, 28, 29
    n-6 polyunsaturated fats, monounsaturated fats and, 28
    saturated fats and, 27, 28
    TFA, 28
    type of fat, 27
  fruit, vegetables, nuts, and, 31
  meat and, 29, 30
  obesity and, 32
  physical activity and, 32
  salt and, 31
Cost-effectiveness, 100, 101
Cross-sectional studies, nutrition research, 6
Curcumin, 79

D
Department of Health, 161
Diet quality indexes (DQIs), 56
Dietary Approaches to Stop Hypertension (DASH) diet, 22, 48, 52, 168
Dietary factors, 130
Dietary fat, CHD and
  fat content of diet, question of, 26
  fish, n–3 polyunsaturated fatty acids, 28, 29
  n-6 polyunsaturated fats, monounsaturated fats and, 28
  saturated fats and, 27, 28
  TFA, 28
  type of fat, 27
Dietary fibers, 131
Dietary for Guidelines Americans (DGA), 162, 170
Dietary guidelines, recommendations for, 170
Dietary patterns
  microbiome, 137–140
  nutrition, 168, 169
Dietary Reference Intakes (DRI), 81, 169
Dietary supplements, 64
  marine fats, 66, 67
  nutrition, 175, 176
  probiotics, 67
  vitamins and minerals
    calcium, 66
    iron, 66
    multivitamins, 64
    vitamin D, 65
Diet-microbiome-metabolite axis
  diet shapes, 133
    amino acids, 135
    bile acids, 133, 135
    short-chain fatty acids, 133, 134
  postbiotics, 135
Digital technologies, 115
  and FOP food labels, 113, 114
Direct-to-consumer (DTC), 121
Disability-adjusted life-years (DALYs), 148
Diversity, 132

E
Eco-labeling, 113
Ecological studies, 7
Ecosystem, 130–131
Energy-adjusted Dietary Inflammatory Index (E-DII), 54
Environmental degradation, 149
Environmental nutrition, 147
Epigallocatechin (EGCG), 77
Epigenome-wide association studies (EWAS), 119
Exposome, 126
Eye diseases, carotenoids, 76

F
Facts Up Front, 111
Fat content of diet, 26
Fatty acids, biosynthesis of, 131–132
Federal Trade Commission (FTC), 160
Fermentable fibers, 131
Finnish Heart Symbol, 111
Fish, 28–29
Flavanols, 77
Flavanones, 78
Flavonoids, 77–78
Flavonols, 78
Food advertising, 100
Food choices, 149
Food corporations
  health posed by, 176, 177
  problem of, 101
Food and Drug Administration's Proposed Label, 109
Food environment, 157

and nutrition policy, 157, 158
industry practices, 158, 159
national nutrition policy, industry influences, 159–162
people's health before profits, 163
Food Guide Pyramid, 170
Food guides, recommendations for, 170, 171
Food labels, recommendations for, 171
back-of-package food labels, 172, 173
front-of-package food labels, 171
Food loss, food waste and, 153–154
Food prices, 99–100
Food processing, microbiome, 137–140
Food production, natural resources and environmental degradation from, 149
Food stamps, 100
Food sustainability, 173
Food swaps, 113
Food synergy, 85, 86
emergence of concept, 87
and disease, 89
healthy and unhealthy dietary patterns, 88
and limitations of epidemiology, 89, 90
meat and health, 89
Mediterranean diet, 87
nutrient deficiency diseases, concept of, 86, 87
Food systems, 146
Food waste, and food loss, 153, 154
Forever chemicals, 178
Fossil fuels, 177
French Paradox, 32
Front-of-package (FOP) food labels, 106
consumer behavior and, 111–113
digital technologies and, 113, 114
diverse types of, 108–110
examples of, 108
history of implementation, 110, 111
nutrition, 171
Fruit, 31

G

Gastrointestinal (GI) tract, 130
Gene-diet interactions, 118–120
Genetic polymorphisms, 122
Genome-wide association studies (GWAS), 119
Genomic-based personalized nutrition (GBPN), 118
applications and testing, 121, 122
challenges of
barriers in practice, 125
current science and research, limitations of, 124, 125
integrating scientific and technological advancements, 126
evidence and progress, 123, 124
gene-diet interactions, 118–120
genomics and nutrition research, 119–121
Genomics, and nutrition research, 119–121
Germ-free animals, 131
Glycans, 136
Government policy, 97
case for action policies, 97
cost-effectiveness, question of, 100, 101
food corporations, problem of, 101
health promotion campaigns, 94
in communities, 94
computer-mediated health promotion, 95
education, advice and encouragement, 96
healthier lifestyle, population adopting, 95, 96
and individual, 95
physician's office, 94, 95
worksite health promotion, 94
nutrition, action policies in, 98
action policies in schools, 98, 99
food advertising, 100
food prices and socioeconomic status, 99, 100
reducing salt content, 98
taxes and subsidies, 99
trans fatty acids, 98
Guideline Daily Amounts, 111

H

Health and Human Services (HHS), 159
Health policy, 126
Health promotion
campaigns, 94
in communities, 94
computer-mediated health promotion, 95
education, advice and encouragement, 96
healthier lifestyle, population adopting, 95, 96
and individual, 95
physician's office, 94, 95
worksite health promotion, 94
limited success of, 173, 174
nutrition policy by governments, 174
strategic plan, 174, 175
Health Star Rating, 111

Healthier lifestyle, population adopting, 95, 96
Health-promoting diet, Western Diet, 49–51
  Asian cultures, diets consumed in, 54, 55
  DASH, 52
  Mediterranean diet, 51, 52
  MIND diet, 53, 54
  Nordic diet, 53
  portfolio diet, 53
Healthy and unhealthy dietary patterns, food synergy, 88
Healthy Hunger Free Kids Act, 160
Healthy volunteer effect, 5
Heart Guide Symbol, 111
Host factors, 132–133
Human gut microbiome
  ecosystem, 130–132
  vitamins and fatty acids, biosynthesis of, 131, 132
Hydroxycinnamic acid, 78
Hyperpalatable, 40, 41, 43
Hypertension, 31

I
Imported foods, 153
Industry practices, 158–159
Infectious diseases, 97
Insertions and deletions (INDELs), 119
Interpretive labels, 112, 114
Iron, 66
Isoflavones, 78

J
Junk food, science in, 161, 162

K
Kaempferol, 78

L
Laparoscopic adjustable gastric banding (LAGB) weight loss, 22
Lectins, 80
Life cycle assessment (LCA), 150, 151
  types of environmental impacts in, 150, 151
Lipidomics, 126
Lipids, microbiome, 136–137
Longitudinal studies, 3
Lutein, 76

M
Marine fats, 66, 67
Marketing, 158, 160, 163
Meat
  and CVD, 29, 30
  food synergy, 89
Mechanistic research, nutrition research, 10
Medical students, and trained doctors, nutrition education for, 176
Mediterranean diet (MD), 22, 33, 39, 51, 52, 168, 181
  food synergy, 87
Mediterranean-Dash Intervention for Neurodegenerative Delay (MIND) diet, 53–54
Mendelian randomization, 119
Meta-analyses, nutrition research, 9, 10
Metabolic-associated diseases, 76
Metabolites, 133, 134
Metabolomics, 126
Microbiome, 130, 180
  characteristics
    diversity, 132
    host factors, 132, 133
    resilience, 132
  dietary patterns and food processing, 137, 140
  diet-microbiome-metabolite axis
    diet shapes, 133–135
    postbiotics, 135
  human gut microbiome
    ecosystem, 130, 131
    vitamins and fatty acids, biosynthesis of, 131, 132
  nutrient-specific modulation of, 135
    carbohydrates, 136
    lipids, 136, 137
    micronutrients, 137
    phytochemicals, 137
    proteins, 136
Micronutrients, microbiome, 137
Minerals
  calcium, 66
  iron, 66
Molecular biology technologies, 121
Monounsaturated fats, 28
Monounsaturated fatty acids, 27
Multiple Traffic Lights, 114
MyPlate, 170

N
n–3 polyunsaturated fatty acids, 28–29
n-6 polyunsaturated fats, 28

National Academies, 176
National nutrition policy, 159–162
 effective regulation, roadblocks to, 159, 160
 junk science, 161, 162
 political power, paying for, 160, 161
Natural resources, 149
Neoliberal theory, 158
Neural tube defects (NTD), 86
New York City Department of Health, 161
Ninth Circuit, 162
Nitrogen-containing compounds, 76, 77
Non-flavonoids, 78–79
Nordic diet, 53
Nordic Keyhole label, 107
NOURISHING, 175
NOVA System, 38, 39
Nutrient deficiency diseases, 86, 87
Nutrient intake, recommendations for, 169
Nutrient metabolism, 130
Nutrient-specific labels shift, 110
Nutriepigenetics, 118
Nutrigenetics, 118
Nutrigenomics, 118
Nutri-Score, 109, 111, 113
Nutrition, 168
 action policies in, 98
  action policies in schools, 98, 99
  food advertising, 100
  food prices and socioeconomic status, 99, 100
  reducing salt content, 98
  taxes and subsidies, 99
  trans fatty acids, 98
 DASH, 168
 dietary guidelines, 170
 dietary patterns, 168, 169
 dietary supplements, 175, 176
 food corporations, health posed by, 176, 177
 food guides, 170, 171
 food labels, 171
  back-of-package food labels, 172, 173
  front-of-package food labels, 171
 health promotion
  limited success of, 173, 174
  policy by governments, 174
  strategic plan, 174, 175
 medical students and trained doctors, nutrition education for, 176
 pseudoscience, 178
  blood types and health, 178, 179
  Bogus weight-loss treatments, 179
  case of Dr Oz, 179
 recommendations for nutrient intake, 169
 sustainable food systems, diets for, 173
 toxic chemicals, suspected danger of, 177, 178
 UPF, 42, 169
Nutrition education, for medical students and trained doctors, 176
Nutrition Facts label, 107, 112, 172
Nutrition policy, 157, 158
 by governments, 174
 industry practices, 158, 159
 national nutrition policy, industry influences, 159
  effective regulation, roadblocks to, 159, 160
  junk science, 161, 162
  political power, paying for, 160, 161
 people's health before profits, 163
Nutrition research, 2
 conflict of interest, problems of, 12
 epidemiological studies, 3
  case-control studies, 5, 6
  cohort studies, 3–5
  cross-sectional studies, 6
  population studies, 7, 8
 evidence, evaluation, 11
 experiments using animals, 10, 11
 mechanistic research, 10
 principles of, 2, 3
 randomized controlled trials, 8
  vs. cohort studies, 8, 9
 systematic reviews and meta-analyses, 9, 10
Nutritional health, and microbiome, 130
 dietary patterns and food processing, 137, 140
 diet-microbiome-metabolite axis, 133–135
 diversity, 132
 host factors, 132, 133
 human gut microbiome, 130–132
 nutrient-specific modulation of, 135–137
 resilience, 132
Nuts, 31

O

Obesity, 15
 causes of, 17–20
 and CHD, 32
 chronic relapsing disease process, 20, 21
 defined and measurement, 16
 prevalence of, 17
 prevention, 21, 22
 treatments, 22, 23
 UPF and, 40–42
Observational, 3

Olive oil, 51
Organosulfur compounds, 79
Organosulfur-containing compounds (OSCs), 79

P
Pesticides, 177
PFAS (polyfluoroalkyl substances), 178
Phenolics, 77
  flavonoids, 77–79
Phthalates, 177
Physical activity, and CHD, 32
Physician's office, health promotion in, 94–95
Phytochemicals, 72, 73, 88, 89, 137, 180
  classifications, food sources and state of evidence, 73
    carotenoids, 73, 76
    cognitive function, 76
    lectins, 80
    metabolic-associated diseases, 76
    nitrogen-containing compounds, 76, 77
    organosulfur compounds, 79
    phenolics, 77–79
  in foods
    and antagonistic effects, 80
    considerations, 81
  microbiome, 137
Phytoestrogens, 78
Phytosterols, 79
Planetary health diet (PHD), 56, 57
Plant-based dietary patterns, 55
Plant-based foods, 152–153
Policymakers, 154
Polyunsaturated fatty acids (PUFA), 27
Population studies, nutrition research, 7, 8
Portfolio diet (PD), 53, 168
Postbiotics, diet-microbiome-metabolite axis, 135
Precision nutrition, GBPN, *see* Genomic-based personalized nutrition (GBPN)
Probiotics, 67
Processed culinary ingredients, 38
Processed foods, 38, 153
Prospective/longitudinal studies, 3
Protective policies, 159
Proteins, microbiome, 136
Proteomics, 126
Pseudoscience, 178
  blood types and health, 178, 179
  Bogus weight-loss treatments, 179
  case of Dr Oz, 179

Q
Quercetin, 78

R
Randomized controlled trials (RCTs), 90
  of bioactive compounds, 72
  vs. cohort studies, 8, 9
  nutrition research, 8
Recommended Dietary Allowances (RDA), 169
Reference intakes, 111
Refined grains, 30
Resilience, 132
Resveratrol, 79

S
Salt
  and CHD/CVD, 31
  reducing, 98
Saturated fats, and CHD, 27–28
Saturated fatty acids (SFA), 27, 33
Seasonal foods, 153
Short-chain fatty acids, diet-microbiome-metabolite axis, 133, 134
Single-nucleotide polymorphisms (SNPs), 119
Smart Choices Program, 163
Societal demands, 149
Socioeconomic status, 99–100
Specific proposed levels (SPL), 81
Sponsoring community organizations, 161
Stilbenes, 79
Strategic plan, 174–175
Suboptimal diet, 118
Subsidies, 99
Sugar, 30
Sugar-sweetened beverages (SSBs), 33
Supermarket, 158–159, 163
Supplemental Nutrition Assistance Program (SNAP), 159, 161
Sustainability metrics and assessment, 150
  greenhouse gas emissions, 151
  LCA, types of environmental impacts in, 150, 151
  life cycle assessment, 150
Sustainable food systems, diets for, 146
  animal-based *vs.* plant-based foods, 152, 153
  approaches for, 151, 152
  challenges for, 149
    adverse nutrition and health outcomes, 150

natural resources and environmental degradation, 149
societal demands, 149
diet, health, and environment, 148
environmental nutrition, 147
food systems, 146
food waste and food loss, 153, 154
imported vs seasonal foods, 153
nutrition, 173
processed *vs.* whole foods, 153
sustainability metrics and assessment, 150
greenhouse gas emissions, 151
LCA, types of environmental impacts in, 150, 151
life cycle assessment, 150
sustainable and healthy diets, foods for, 152
Systematic reviews, nutrition research, 9, 10

T
Tannins, 79
Taxes, 99
Tea, and CHD/CVD, 31, 32
Total cholesterol (TC), 26, 33
Toxic chemicals, suspected danger of, 177, 178
Trade promotion fees, 158
Traditional Balanced Korean diet, 54
Traditional Japanese diet, 55
Trans fatty acids (TFA), 28, 86
removal of, 98

U
U.S. Department of Agriculture (USDA), 170
Ultra-processed foods (UPF), 18, 38, 169
and disease, 40
and nutrition advice, 42
and obesity, 40–42
dietary recommendations, 38, 39
Unhealthy food consumption, 106
Unhealthy processed foods, 158
United States Department of Agriculture (USDA), 159
Unprocessed/minimally processed foods, 38

V
Vegetables, 31
Vegetarian diets, 55, 56
Visceral fat deposits, 16
Vitamin
biosynthesis of, 131–132
multivitamins, 64
vitamin D, 65
Vitamin D, 65

W
Western diet, 149, 168
and global health, 47–51
health and environmental sustainability
PHD, 56, 57
vegetarian diets, 55, 56
health-promoting diet, 49–51
Asian cultures, diets consumed in, 54, 55
DASH, 52
Mediterranean diet, 51, 52
MIND diet, 53, 54
Nordic diet, 53
portfolio diet, 53
Whole foods, 153
Whole grains, 30
Worksite health promotion, 94

Z
Za Srce, 111
Zeaxanthin, 76

GPSR Compliance

The European Union's (EU) General Product Safety Regulation (GPSR) is a set of rules that requires consumer products to be safe and our obligations to ensure this.

If you have any concerns about our products, you can contact us on ProductSafety@springernature.com

In case Publisher is established outside the EU, the EU authorized representative is:

Springer Nature Customer Service Center GmbH
Europaplatz 3
69115 Heidelberg, Germany

Batch number: 10505321

Printed by Printforce, the Netherlands